WOMEN'S ANATOMY *of* AROUSAL

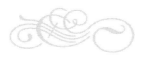

SECRET MAPS TO BURIED PLEASURE

SHERI WINSTON

CNM, RN, BSN, LMT

Anatomy and Occasional Other Illustrations by the Author

MANGO GARDEN

About The Intimate Arts Center

SHERI WINSTON'S INTIMATE ARTS CENTER is dedicated to providing empowering, enriching and entertaining erotic education.

We envision a world where sex is understood, honored and free from shame, where our bodies' ecstatic potential is explored and celebrated, and relationships are based on integrity, compassion and love.

The Center offers online intimate arts classes and courses, books, an e-newsletter, blog posts and more.

Mango Garden Press is our publishing imprint. Our books are available in physical form and on Kindle. An Audible audiobook version of *Women's Anatomy of Arousal* is also available.

Services include speeches and presentations, and consultations and counseling for individuals and couples (both phone-based and in person).

To sign up for our newsletter, purchase other products, get more information about sponsoring or booking Sheri Winston, or to learn more, please visit us at our website: INTIMATEARTSCENTER.COM.

©2010 Sheri Winston / Mango Garden Press
COVER DESIGN: Sherry Williams/Oxygen Design
INTERIOR DESIGN: Tilman Reitzle
COVER PHOTOGRAPH: Amanda Giles

ISBN: 978-0578-033952

Library of Congress # 2009937322

V_10

MANGO GARDEN PRESS
PO BOX 3184, KINGSTON, NY, 12402
WWW.MANGOGARDENPRESS.COM

Testimonials
Discover Why Sex Experts Are Saying:

"What I especially love about Women's Anatomy of Arousal is that it's fun, funny and packed with fabulous information. Guaranteed to inspire and enhance your love life! The book has a fantastic collection of illustrations, the likes of which I have not seen before. Sheri Winston is a delightful and creative sex educator."

ANNIE SPRINKLE, PH.D.—*Sex-ecologist, Artist, Author,* Dr. Sprinkle's Spectacular Sex

"I am a sex educator and author and I couldn't believe all the information that I learned from this book. Sheri Winston is a very talented genius. If you really want to know how to arouse a woman, then I highly recommend this book. If you are a woman, plain and simple then you should buy this book right now—there's a whole world of pleasure yet to discover and this book provides the keys!"

JAIYA—*New World Sex Education, Author,* Red Hot Touch—A Head-to-Toe Handbook for Mind Blowing Orgasms

"Winston is an amazing, articulate, accessible teacher. Her book takes you on a joyous and illuminating journey into empowerment and ecstatic awareness."

LASARA FIREFOX ALLEN, MPNLP—*Creator of Gratitude Games and Author,* Sexy Witch

"For more than 20 years I have been an ardent student of sexuality, sexual energy and sexual pleasure. I can say without hesitation and all enthusiasm that this is THE BEST BOOK I HAVE EVER READ ON WOMEN'S SEXUALITY—bar none. Sheri's voice comes through on every page—brilliantly, comfortingly, soothingly, encouragingly, tauntingly, lovingly. Thank you, Sheri, for your gift to women and the world."

PAT PARISI—*Sex Educator, Sexuality & Relationship Counselor, Retreat Facilitator, Healer*

"Brings our recognition of the depth and subtleties of feminine anatomy out of the fog and into the 21st Century. This one-of-a-kind revolutionary new book should be required reading for every woman (and her partner) with a true desire to take her pleasure to the next level . . . and beyond!"

PATRICIA TAYLOR, PH.D.—*Author,* Expanded Orgasm and Expand Her Orgasm Tonight!

"Useful, intelligent sex education requires clear explanations about how sensual pleasure and procreation are connected. Sheri Winston's book is a monumental step in that direction—and a wonderful gift to the world!"

RICHARD ANTON DIAZ—*Founder of Sexy Spirits and Taontric Massage*

"Winston is one of the most interesting, engaging and unique sex educators out there. Her work in book form is as riveting as her live workshops. Whether you're a man or a woman, you'll definitely learn something new. I know I did!"

JAMYE WAXMAN, M.ED.—*Author,* Getting Off: A Woman's Guide to Masturbation

"This easy-to-read, enlightening book is like a good novel, a good friend, a big sister and a knowledgeable, understanding lover rolled into one! It's packed with information your health professional could never explain with such ease or detail."

CARLYLE JANSEN—*Sex educator and founder,* Good for Her sexuality boutique

"Winston has a unique ability to convey information about anatomy and physiology in playful and accessible terms. Essential reading for women and those who love them."

MARK A. MICHAELS and PATRICIA JOHNSON—*Authors of* The Essence of Tantric Sexuality and Tantra for Erotic Empowerment Acknowledgments

Acknowledgments

FIRST AND FOREMOST, I THANK my love, Carl Frankel. Many authors acknowledge to their partners that they "couldn't have done it without you," but in this case, it is quite literally true. Without his writing expertise, editing skill, organizational wizardry and vision of excellence and beauty, this book would not be what it is. Carl, you are a brilliant wordsmith, an exacting editor and a wise counselor. Your fortitude and dedication to making this dream a reality have buoyed me through this arduous birth. Many contributed to this book's incarnation. I am immeasurably grateful to Tilman Reitzle. I also thank Cindy Spitzer, Amanda Giles (cover photo), Sherry Williams (Oxygen Design), Val Vadeboncoeur, Constance Angelo and Ed Butler.

Over the years, many people have supported the vision of Wholistic Sexuality. I am deeply grateful to everyone who's sponsored workshops, hosted classes and sponsored events over the years. . Gratitude goes out to all—space constraints don't allow me to thank each of you, but your generosity and support are much appreciated.

I am especially indebted to The Federation of Feminist Women's Health Centers and their book *A New View of a Woman's Body*, which opened my eyes to the realization that our contemporary female genital anatomy models are inaccurate and incomplete. That book started me on my 'hunt for buried pleasure' and is the basis of many parts of my paradigm.

I am deeply grateful for the support and love of my friends. I thank my many teachers and mentors in the healing and birthing arts, including every woman who birthed with me or came to me for care, for helping me learn what's true and see the natural wonder of birth.

Cory, my son, thank you for choosing to get born to me! Thanks to my family for your love!

Yummy juicy thanks to my intimate partners—deliciously sexy, brilliant and devoted learners of the erotic and relationship arts. Special appreciation, love and gratitude to Scott, my 'wusband' and learning partner of twenty years. And special thanks to sweeties Rob, Brian and Gary.

If I've neglected to mention anyone else who contributed directly to the book or to my wonderful life, please accept my apologies. It reflects a failure of memory, not a lack of appreciation.

Finally, I again want to thank my life partner and beloved consort, Carl. While this book would not be what it is without you, more importantly, my life would not be what it is without you. Beloved, I am so glad, so very glad that you have come.

THIS BOOK IS DEDICATED to the bold and the brave who take the risk of questioning the status quo; to the pioneers and visionaries who see beyond the scrim; and to the adventurers who explore the edges, seek treasure and bring back riches for our enlightenment.

TABLE OF CONTENTS

Section One

Maps, Models and Mistakes

Section Two

Journey to the Origin of the World

Section Three

Becoming an Erotic Virtuoso

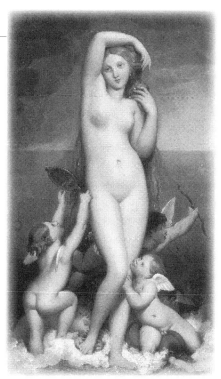

A Woman Waits for Me
(excerpt)

BY WALT WHITMAN

*A woman waits for me,
she contains all, nothing is lacking,
Yet all were lacking if sex were lacking,
or if the moisture of the right man were lacking.*

*Sex contains all, bodies, souls,
meanings, proofs, purities,
delicacies, results, promulgations,
songs, commands, health, pride,
the maternal mystery, the seminal milk,
all hopes, benefactions, bestowals,
all the passions, loves, beauties, delights of the earth,
all the governments, judges, gods,
follow'd persons of the earth,*

*These are contain'd in sex as parts of itself
and justifications of itself.*

*Without shame the man I like knows and avows
the deliciousness of his sex,
Without shame the woman I like
knows and avows hers.*

Section One

Maps, Models and Mistakes

*"We don't see things as they are,
we see things as we are."*

ANAIS NIN, *taken from the Talmud*

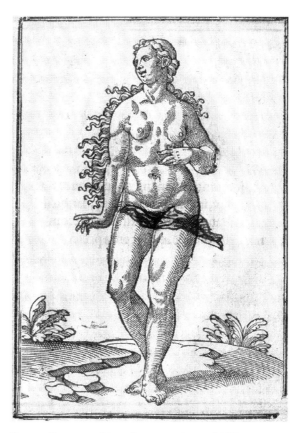

JEHAN COUSIN—*Livre de pourtraiture, 1608*

CHAPTER ONE

Sex, Sex, Sex— It's All About Sex

"Sex lies at the root of life, and we can never learn to reverence life until we know how to understand sex."

HAVELOCK ELLIS

Greetings!

MY NAME IS SHERI WINSTON, and I'll be taking you on an in-depth, illustrated tour of the land of female genitalia, feminine sexuality and the intimate erotic arts. Whether you're a man or a woman, the information in these pages can help you have great sex, so long as you have female parts or like to play with them.

I'll begin with a love story that may just be the grandest love story of all. It comes from the Hindu tradition.

The Love Song of Shakti and Shiva

In the beginning was the One. The One was all and everything, and for eons it reveled in being One for millennia of magnificent unitary bliss. Over the course of unimaginable time, however, the One grew bored. (Even the Divine gets bored with itself eventually.)

So the One split into two. One part was Shakti—she of energy, flow, and movement. The other was Shiva—he of consciousness, presence, and purpose.

As soon as the one became two, they gazed upon each other, fell madly in love, and wanted nothing more than to re-unite. They clasped each other passionately and explored all the ways two could merge into one. They entered each other and dissolved the boundaries between them. For millennia they made love, exquisite erotic love. At long last they again achieved oneness as they exploded in mutual simultaneous orgasm.

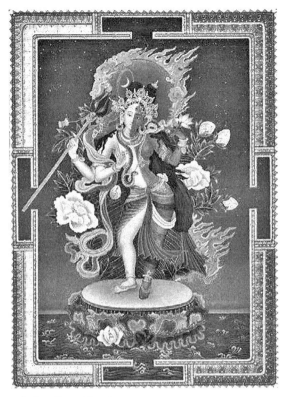

Shakti Shiva Thanka

In that moment, the entire universe was born. All life sprang into being and is springing still. It was the original big bang!

The story of Shakti and Shiva is an origin story about the universe, and a story about each and every one of us. Like them, we long for connection, are magnetized by attraction, and drawn by the desire to merge into oneness. Like them, passion is what connects us to all life, and desire is our path to divine union.

Sex—The Essential Life Force

The saga of Shakti and Shiva reminds us that ecstasy is our birthright and the source of all existence. It also tells us that sex is more than our individual desires, erotic experiences, intimate connections and sexual behavior. It is the deepest expression of the power of creation. The mating drive is one of the most powerful forces in our world: it has to be or we wouldn't be here, gloriously alive amid the wondrous diversity and complexity of existence. Asexual reproduction was a great starter plan for Earth, but it takes the desire to mate and mingle genes to birth the unimaginable and wondrous biodiversity of our world. Sex is the basic urge to merge.

Your individual sexuality is your small piece of that primal power—the vital, pulsing life force. Your sexuality connects to that cosmic energy: they are one and the same thing, only on the micro and macro levels.

How you relate to that immense power has a pervasive impact on your life. You can repress your sexuality. You can go "repression light" and downplay it. Or, you can take the other road and . . . *celebrate* it! Your sexuality can take you on a sacred ecstatic path that unites you profoundly to all life throughout time. At the end of the day, the choice is yours. You can learn to fully and consciously open the inner portal to your sexual

> *"Sexual love is the most stupendous fact of the universe, and the most magical mystery our poor blind senses know."*
>
> AMY LOWELL

life force, and in so doing gain access to divine bliss and link to your uninhibited wild power. That exquisite connection to the cosmos—the *erotic* cosmos—resides inside you, right there in your sexy center.

If sex were merely the natural mating behavior of putting Tab A into Slot B, everyone would be good at it. But sex isn't just about who we do and how we do them, and it isn't only about the ways we get aroused and orgasmic, either. Your sexuality goes to the heart of who you are. All of your relationships, not just your actively sexual ones, grow from this root.

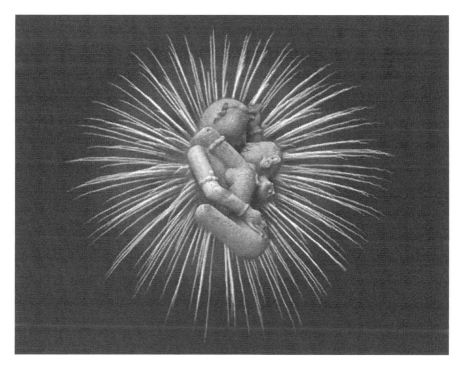

SHERI WINSTON—*Shakti and Shiva Making Love*

When I say "all of your relationships," I mean that literally...including your most significant connection of all, your relationship with yourself. If you want to have better sex and more satisfying intimate relationships, the place to begin is with yourself—and, more specifically, with your relationship to your own sexuality.

The Learning Animal

The more you understand who you are sexually and how you operate, the better you'll do in all aspects of your life, sex included. There's no question that sex is a natural behavior, which for most animals means an automatic "acting out" of their breeding blueprint. But we are humans— a very fancy sort of animal indeed—with special, big, malleable brains. We are *the learning animal*. As such, each of us is the result of a complex interplay between a long slow evolutionary process and our local and unique influences and environment. Not only are you the *result* of a dance between biology and culture, you *are* a dance between biology and culture! You entwine nature and nurture; you weave together what is inborn with what you've learned. All these forces and factors together create your own unique sexuality. Know thyself—learn about thyself!— and you'll know how to access your ecstasy.

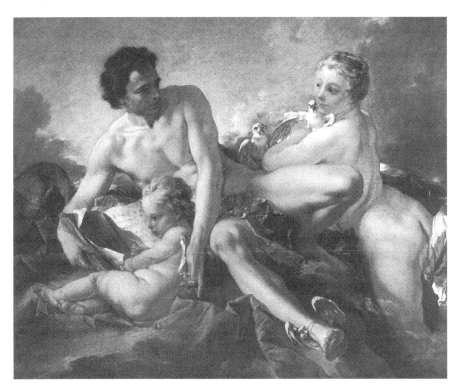

François Boucher—*Education of Cupid*

WOMEN'S ANATOMY OF AROUSAL

Hardware and Software

When I tell people I'm a sex teacher, I sometimes get this response: "Sex is natural! I don't need a teacher for that." This is both true and not true.

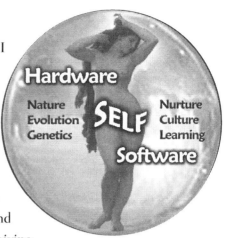

SHERI WINSTON—*Hardware and Software*

In some ways, humans are like computers. We come equipped with hardware, the factory-installed equipment we were born with. The forces of nature shaped evolution and produced our unique DNA blueprint, giving us blue eyes or brown skin. It also hardwired us with certain types of sexual behavior. We all know about the basic mammalian humping motion, for instance. This isn't something we learned at school, and we didn't need Nike to inspire us, either. We just do it.

We're not just our hardwiring, though. We also come loaded with lots of software—our extensive programming, also known as culturally learned behavior. We probably do more learning than any other species. Much of our sexuality is learned, absorbed throughout our lifetime as we simmered in the soup of culture. We learn from our culture how to kiss and caress, what's acceptable and what's taboo, what's hot and what's not.

In other words, sex is natural *and* we learn sex. And you know what? If it's learnable, then we can learn to get better at it. We can unlearn bad habits and acquire new skills, whether the activity in question is scuba diving, speaking a foreign language, or sex. While it's true that people bring varying levels of aptitude to what they do, we all have what it takes to get more skilled at the erotic arts. Our software is made for upgrading.

If you're one of those people who thinks that sex is something you do, not something you learn, I invite you to reconsider that view. It's only partially correct and not especially useful. Why corral your potential unnecessarily? If you believe your sexual status quo is all that's possible, then that's all you'll ever have. But if you believe that you can develop erotic mastery, then that's what you'll achieve, so long as your faith is accompanied by commitment and skilled guidance.

We're all on a lifelong learning journey. By making sex a conscious part of it, you can make your whole life better—filled with more pleasure, power and connection.

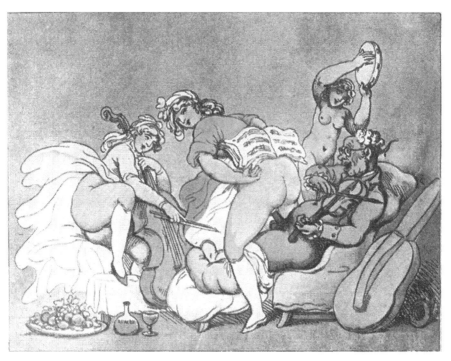

THOMAS ROWLANDSON—*The Concert, c. 1800*

The Planet of Missing Information

This book builds on a framework I've developed called Wholistic Sexuality, an empowering vision of healthy, loving, responsible, respectful and ecstatic sexuality. Wholistic Sexuality honors the wisdom of ancient sex-positive societies, incorporates modern scientific research and embraces the mind-body-spirit-heart connection. Anatomy matters—anatomy matters a lot!—but at the end of the day, great sex is about much more than physiology.

> *"You never change things by fighting the existing reality. To change something, build a new model that makes the old model obsolete."*
>
> **BUCKMINSTER FULLER**

One of the foundational premises of Wholistic Sexuality is that, if we want to fulfill our erotic potential, we need accurate models to guide us. Unfortunately, in our culture, our sexual atlas has lots of missing pages, and a lot of the maps that do exist are just plain wrong. We're especially challenged in our understanding of women, including both the specifics of female anatomy and more immaterial concepts such as feminine energy and power. Realistic, helpful models of female sexuality are not easy to come by (so to speak), hence the focus of this book.

It's hard to believe that in this day and age, so much basic information about female genital anatomy is missing from our science, our media and our minds. Yes, we know there's "stuff" down there, but the remarkable truth is that our contemporary models of female genitalia are incomplete and inaccurate. Many of the structures responsible for arousal and orgasm are absent from our models or woefully misunderstood, forcing women and their lovers to look for that legendary mega-orgasmic place without a good map to guide them. This book provides the model you've been missing. Here, you'll find the map you need to fully realize female sexual potential, whether it's yours, your partner's or both.

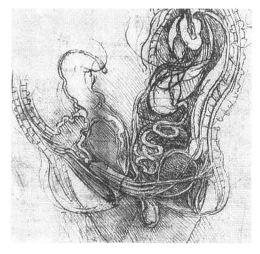

LEONARDO DA VINCI—*Studies of the Sexual Act, 1519*

The heart (or perhaps crotch) of the book focuses on women's sexual anatomy, including all the parts women have (including the obscure ones) and how they work together as an integrated system. Women have an interconnected network of structures that act in concert to choreograph arousal and orgasm.

Sadly, though, many women don't know about their whole set of equipment. And if that's the case for women, who after all own the apparatus, it's doubly so for men!

If this is your situation, don't feel bad. Very few people know about these parts or understand how they enable both reproduction and erotic ecstasy. I'm not just referring to "lay" people here. Many professionals, including sex teachers and gynecologists, don't have accurate or complete maps, either.

If you're like most women, you're using only part of your genital equipment to generate the music of stimulation, dance the path of arousal, and ride the waves of your orgasmic potential. Now, it's true that you don't need the entire system to have compelling erotic experiences. But when you work with and master the entire arousal system, you'll experience every orgasmic cliché there is, and maybe discover some new ones, too. You, too, can be an erotic virtuoso!

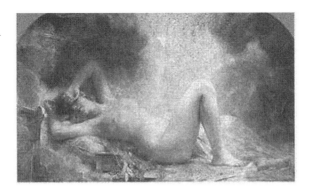

LEON COMERRE—
*Danae and
the Shower
of Gold*

What do I mean by this? I mean that you can learn to get turned on wonderfully quickly when you choose to, and easily achieve states of deep arousal. You can expand the kinds of stimulation that arouse you to the point that it doesn't matter much if your partner is sucking on your pinkie or your clitoris—either way, it makes you wild. In addition, you can provide your partner with over-the-top pleasure, not only due to your technical skills but also because pleasuring him or her turns you on so much! (That's right, you can get off and even come from getting your sweetie off!)

Last and definitely not least, you can achieve mastery in the wide, wild and wonderful world of orgasm. You can be multi-orgasmic, mega-orgasmic and much more-gasmic. All this awaits you through the information in this book.

The Luscious Land of Arousal and Orgasm

Expertise in arousal and orgasm is where erotic virtuosity begins. So let's begin with a brief exploration of these realms.

Sexual arousal is an altered state of consciousness. An altered state is any mind-body mode that operates differently from our everyday awareness and transcends ordinary consciousness. Dreaming is one such state. Meditation and daydreaming are others. And, did you know that women actually need to enter an altered state to successfully labor and birth?

> *"An orgasm a day
> keeps the doctor away."*
>
> MAE WEST

When we get turned on, we enter a state of non-ordinary reality. The arousal trance is characterized by deep awareness of bodily sensation, a decrease in pain perception and often a feeling of timelessness. Our heightened pleasure can produce euphoria and ecstasy. Our heart races, our breath quickens, and we become absorbed and entranced. Self-consciousness evaporates and a feeling of relaxed concentration takes over. When you're aroused, you don't need to plan or think. The arousal itself becomes your guide: you simply go where it takes you.

Arousal also draws us into an intense focus on our immediate physical and emotional experience. We become acutely aware of our senses; our mindscape overflows with sensational sensation. Our mundane daily existence can be left far behind as we soar into the realm of the ecstatic.

Arousal alters our perception of both pain and pleasure. During arousal, we become increasingly and exquisitely sensitive to pleasure. At the same time, our ability to perceive pain diminishes, causing varying levels of analgesia. This accounts for the experience of a sensation that only minutes ago was irritating, painful, or simply not arousing now giving intense pleasure. In arousal, the fine line between pleasure and pain is constantly shifting, yet another reason why partners need to be in constant communication about what is and isn't working.

Although the capacity for arousal is something we're all born with, we can learn to deepen our arousal trance while expanding the pathways that lead us into this blissful altered state of consciousness. The more we allow ourselves to surrender to the trance, and the more we cultivate the practices that bring us there, the more we'll find ourselves having the transcendent sex we dream of.

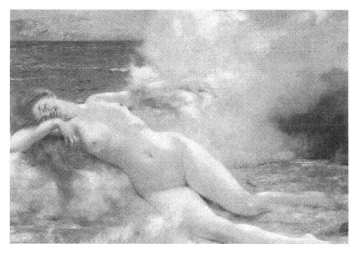

HENRI GERVEX—*The Birth of Venus, 1896*

CLIMBING THE AROUSAL STAIRCASE

Arousal is a journey into enchantment, a trip into a dramatically altered state of being. The process of arousal can be likened to climbing a set of stairs composed of ten steps. The ground floor is ordinary reality. As we

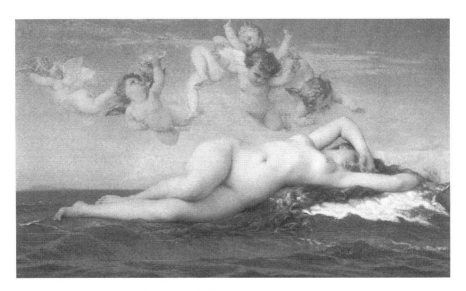

start to get slightly turned on, we ascend to the first step, and as our arousal increases, up we go. We can only ascend one step at a time, though. We can't soar from the ground floor to the top step in one giant leap. We require the stimulus of a physiological feedback loop to propel us to the next level of arousal, and so we need to proceed from step to step consecutively. We can learn how to climb the steps quickly, and, conversely, how to slow down and linger on a step, deepening each level of the journey.

This ten-step arousal process can most accurately be thought of as having three separate phases of three steps each, plus a very special tenth step. We can think of the first three steps as early arousal, the middle three as medium-level arousal, and the last three as high-level arousal. As for the tenth step, well, that one is a doozy. It's the one we get to once lift-off is complete and we've settled into orgasmic orbit. It's where we ride the wave of our orgasms.

To a significant degree, what happens while we're in orbit remains within our control. We can shape our orgasmic experience with our intention, breath, sound and movement. In fact, we can use these sex skills to keep climbing!

I heartily recommend that you don't make getting to the tenth step your priority, although it's great to be able to get there quickly when you want. In fact, I suggest that you make a habit of playing around on the stairs for quite a while. Arousal trance states have depth—either more or less, depending on how much time you spend dallying at each phase. The deeper you get into your trance, the better. The more totally immersed you become in any one particular step of arousal, the easier it will be to get to the next level, and it will also be less likely that you'll get distracted or jarred back down the stairs. The longer you build arousal, the more energy you'll have to ride and play with. The more rapt you are in your own rapture, the more spectacular your peak experience will be.

THE VARIETIES OF ORGASMIC EXPERIENCE

I used to believe that there was basically only one type of orgasmic experience. This was consistent with the usual formal definition of orgasm as a short-lived genital experience consisting of successive waves of pleasurable spasms. This characterization positions orgasm as a climactic event—in other words, a finale. And it's true, that's often what it is for people (almost always for guys, and frequently for women). But orgasm can be much more than that:

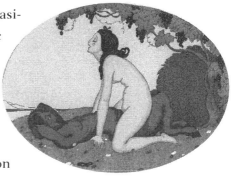

GERDA WEGENER—*Satyr, c. 1900*

- It can be wave upon wave of ecstasy lasting many minutes. You can get to a place where you stay in a general state of orgasm, rising and falling, cresting into the pleasure over and over again.

- You can experience orgasm in any part of your body, or in any of your energy centers or chakras.*

- You can have orgasms that include only part of your genitals (your clitoris, for instance) or ones that include every yummy bit of your equipment.

- Your orgasm can transport you to an experience of yourself as divine.

- It can take the form of a shared love-gasm, centered in your heart and the heart of your Beloved. (In fact, any of these experiences can be experienced alone or with a partner.)

When you become an erotic virtuoso, you can learn to come easily and often. You can also become an adventurer, let's call it an "orgasmonaut," exploring the vast realms of orgasmic experiences.

---

* Chakras are energy centers or vortexes located in our energetic body. Although western medicine is skeptical of their existence, they are foundational to the eastern healing traditions.

The Altered States of Orgasmia

Here's a short list (okay, not so short a list!) of types of orgasm I've experienced:

- Little tickly genital-sneeze orgasms

- Big ones, bigger ones, and even bigger ones

- Megagasms (ridiculously huge ones that seem to go on forever)

- Multi-multi-multi-gasms

- Laugh-gasms

- Sob-gasms

- Love-gasms

- Chakra-gasms

- Releasing waves of flowing, "surrender" (or yin) orgasms

- Fierce clutching, driving (yang) orgasms

- Mini-orgasms and "aftershocks" (known as *kriyas* in the tantric tradition)

- Energy orgasms ranging from small shuddery ones to huge body-wracking ones

- Orgasms centered in different body parts and sex centers: mouth, throat, heart, breasts and nipples, clitoris, pussy, uterus, ass.

- Full-body orgasms

- Projectile, squirting, gushing orgasms (orgasms with female ejaculation)

- Surprise orgasms that sneak up on you

- Telepathic mutual mind-blowers when you feel you're in perfect intuitive union with your partner.

If I've had these orgasms, you can have them, too!

Owning Your Sexual Potential

The information in this book is drawn from many wells: my personal life; decades of work as a midwife, women's healthcare provider, holistic healer and sex teacher; obscure scientific knowledge; modern sexology research; and ancient sacred sexuality traditions. It was a very personal journey that got me where I am today.

This will also be a personal (albeit guided) journey for you. These pages have one purpose only: to facilitate your voyage. You have everything you need to connect to your own power, create relationships centered in love and integrity, and lead an erotically ecstatic life. You are your own gateway, and also your sole authority.

Anyone who's spent much time with doctors knows that while they wear the expert's white coat and sound authoritative, they don't always have the right answers. As a general principle, it's wise to maintain a healthy skepticism about official experts when they tell you about your body and how to do things differently or better.

I firmly believe that it's our duty to question authority. Just because something is in a book or believed by most people doesn't make it true. That goes for this book and this expert, too. I'm claiming that women's genitals have parts that have gone missing in our culture. Here's my expert advice: don't believe me. Instead, check out my claims for yourself, using the laboratory of your own body.

What this means in practice is, don't just read. *Do!* Become an intrepid explorer of your genitals

> *"Do not believe anything because it is said by an authority, or if it is said to come from angels, or from Gods, or from an inspired source. Believe it only if you have explored it in your own heart and mind and body and found it to be true."*
>
> **BUDDHA**

and sexual potential. Be a junior scientist and gather your own data. Once you've done this, you'll *really* know the truth, not because an authority or book told you, but because you experienced it directly.

More Than Sex

I applaud you for your courage in picking up this book. Good for you (and your partners, too!). I'm sure that, at a minimum, you did so because you want to give and get more sexual pleasure and enjoy more fulfilling erotic relationships. But this book isn't only about how to have better sex. It's also about deepening your connection to yourself, accessing more joy in all aspects of your life, having sustainable, authentic, and joyous intimate relationships, and feeling fabulous about yourself. This is about choosing happiness, reveling in your freedom, and experiencing your divinity—all through the gateway of your sexuality.

Imagine what it would be like if your sexuality were integrated with your whole being—your amazing mind, your wondrous body, your loving heart, and your sacred spirituality. Picture yourself able to honor your passions, revel in pleasure, and delight in your sexuality. Envision yourself as a truly free being able to choose healthy relationships that support your most empowered life. Imagine loving your body . . . *totally*. Take a moment to see yourself, alone or with a Beloved, in a beautiful temple where sex is a sacrament that celebrates your erotic desires as a divine connection to all. Can you see it? Do you want it? It's yours for the claiming.

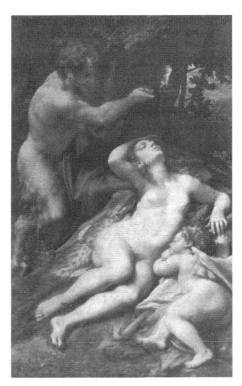

"Of the delights of this world, man cares most for sexual intercourse, yet he has left it out of his heaven."

MARK TWAIN

A Note About Language

As discussed in greater detail elsewhere in this book, our culture hasn't given us a good vocabulary for talking about sex. We have scientific terms ("vagina," "penis"), baby talk ("tushy" and "wee-wee"), euphemisms ("down there"), and super-charged so-called dirty words like (and, yes, I'm about to say them) "pussy" and "fuck."

ANTONIO CORREGGIO—*Venus and Cupid with a Satyr*

These last words and others of that ilk shock and offend so much they're banned from radio and television. Yet they're just words, just a collection of sounds and syllables that we collectively agree have a certain meaning. They only mean what we make them mean, and they're only "dirty" when we make them so.

As a healer, teacher and writer, I constantly have to navigate the straits of the limitations of our language. It's not easy to do: the choice is essentially between formal to the point of pomposity (scientific language), vague and silly (baby words and euphemisms), and provocative (the "dirty words"). I've dealt with this by being varied in my usage. Sometimes I've gone with the clinical term or my own personal variations on them. Occasionally I opt for terms from Sanskrit, the holy language of ancient India—using "yoni" for the female genitalia and "lingam" for the penis—which have the blessing of being sacred and the disadvantage of not being widely understood.

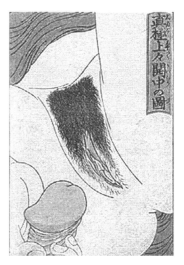

Utagawa Kunisada—*Japan*

And I also use juicier language.

When I've taken the latter course, it hasn't been to shock or offend. It has, though, been a conscious choice, and, in a sense, a political act. The simple truth is that we need a more straightforward, comfortable way to talk about sex than our current language provides. One way to do this is by taking the charge off words that currently titillate or offend. When I use "fuck" or "pussy," I do so for two reasons. First, they're straightforward and descriptive (and often sexy, fun and lighthearted). Second, by treating them as if they have no charge, it helps to normalize them.

Some years ago, Eve Ensler's *Vagina Monologues* took the V-word out of the gutter and made vaginas respectable. At some point, hopefully in the not-too-distant future, "pussy" and other so-called dirty words will be equally legitimate and benign.

One final note about language: When I use the terms 'women' and 'female' in reference to anatomy, I'm referring to the genitalia of people who are born with a vagina, uterus and erectile network. Usually these will be cis-women. ('Cis' means your gender identity matches the sex you were assigned at birth.) Some trans men have a vagina and erectile network. The anatomy in this book is accurate for them. However, this book does not include the varieties of surgically-created genitals that trans women may have. That is not because I don't value all bodies and all genitals (I very much do), but because it is beyond the scope of this book and of my expertise.

The Most Fun Homework, Ever

This book is divided into three sections and twelve chapters:

- The first section (*Maps, Models and Mistakes*) lays the foundation for the material that follows. Consisting of four chapters, it examines our confused cultural view of sexuality, lays out the transformative Wholistic Sexuality framework, and delves into ancient Taoist wisdom as a way of understanding our sexuality.

- The second section (*Journey to the Origin of the World*) is also made up of four chapters. It addresses everything you wanted to know (and probably didn't know to ask) about female genitalia.

- The third and final section (*Becoming an Erotic Virtuoso*) guides you in taking what you've learned in the first two sections and using it to achieve your full sexual potential. It includes a chapter especially for men.

*"I'm such a good lover because
I practice a lot on my own."*

WOODY ALLEN

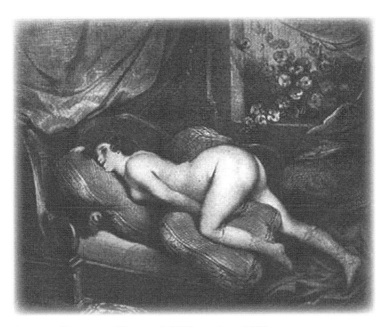

ACHILLE DEVERIA—*Woman Self-Pleasuring, 1857*

This book includes an array of suggestions of experiential things to do. Call the activities games, exercises, practices, rituals, or whatever works for you. Needless to say, you don't have to do anything I tell you. (I'm not your mother and you don't listen to her, anyway!). I invite you to check out each suggestion. If it sounds good, try it! Think of these ideas as a smorgasbord, a banquet of choices. Feel free to take what appeals to you and leave the rest. Try some new options that you haven't tasted before, or check back later and see if your desires have changed. These are serving suggestions, not orders.

There is a great deal of visual material in this book. I encourage you to spend time with it. Doing so will deepen your understanding of female genitalia while also providing insight into how various cultures have distorted our understanding of the female body.

Just looking isn't enough, though. If you don't actually view, feel, touch, and play with the equipment, you'll be less likely to discover your pathways and potential.

Yes, that's right. Women, I just told you to go play with yourself and I meant it! Men, you're welcome to help, if your goddess so desires. Be hands-on . . . literally!

In fact, if you really want to "get it," you will need to both experience and witness the transformations of arousal. These changes will help you to fully understand what's there, how it works, and how to make it really happy.

Specifically, here's what I recommend. While you read the anatomy chapters, play along by checking out everything on your own (or a female friend's) body . . . with her consent, of course! Almost all the structures I discuss can easily be felt, and most can be seen.

Start when you or your female partner are not aroused, and then feel and see the structures again at different levels of arousal. It will soon be eminently clear to you that this book's description of female genitalia is accurate. Plus, it makes doing your homework a whole lot of fun. In fact, we should probably call it homeplay, because it's definitely not work!

Women, I suggest that you take the tour alone the first time. If you are partnered, make a second trip to introduce your lover to the wonders of your body.

To make your learning experience fun and easy, we've made liberal use of sidebars, some of which run throughout the book. There are five running sidebars in all:

GUIDED TOUR

*S*tep-by-step instructions for the female genital tour. Follow them to get the most out of your homeplay sexploration.

Owner's Manual

Greater detail about gynecological health issues that women will find especially useful.

GODDESS GUIDE

Ways women can honor and connect to the spiritual power of their bodies and sexuality.

Play and Practice

Activities, exercises, games and suggestions to help develop your erotic skills and have more fun playing with yourself.

HOT TIPS FOR GUYS

These sidebars are designed to help men understand how to honor, humor, handle and please the wondrous pussy and the women who own them. Men, if you just want the essentials, check out these sidebars and the short concluding chapter.

Whether you're a man or a woman, I encourage you to enter this book in a spirit of adventure, with optimism and an open mind. Why accept cultural canards about sex when you can experience the amazing reality? Why wait any longer to expand your repertoire of what's possible? Thank you for embarking on this journey toward your very own authentic, sexiest self.

CHAPTER TWO

A Tale of Cultural Confusion

"All 'Eros' is custom . . . any sexual act is moral or immoral by precisely the same laws of morality as any other human act; all other rules about sex are simply customs—local and transient. There are more codes of sexual customs then a dog has fleas—and all they have in common is that they are 'ordained by God'."

ROBERT A. HEINLEIN

Mixed Messages

BECAUSE OF ITS ENORMOUS PRIMAL POWER, sex has always presented a major challenge for human societies. All cultures throughout time have recognized that the sex drive can't be left to run utterly wild. In sex-positive cultures, desire is celebrated in sacred containers of ritual and ceremony that channel the power of fertility and creation magic. Sex-negative cultures take the opposite tack. They control the sex drive with inflexible laws, constrict with repressive beliefs and viciously punish transgression. All cultures have contained or managed that wildness one way or another. Our culture is no different.

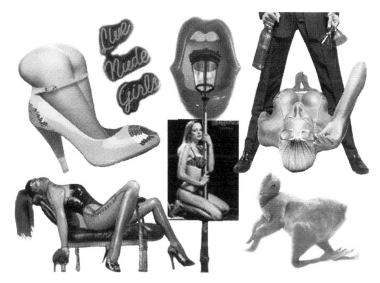

SHERI WINSTON—*Modern Sex*

No one is neutral about sex. Everyone has strong opinions, feelings, beliefs and values. We come to these attitudes in large part through our culture. Whatever our personal situation may be and however together we are (or not) regarding our sexuality, one fact is true for us all: our culture is obsessed and confused about sex.

Let's start with the obsessed part. Sexual images and ideas are plastered everywhere. We are constantly told that sexiness and desirability are paramount, and sold a veneer of sexual wildness.

The visual images that accompany this onslaught are as predictable as they are limiting. We're shown slender, curvy bodies, occupying a fantasy world where everyone is young (or looks young) and beauty is defined by an unrealistic photoshopped standard.

Now for the mixed-up part. Along with all the overt messages about how cool it is to be young and hip, and how hot it is to look and act sexy, we get a contrary and more covert message that tells us actual sex is shameful and embarrassing. The inference is that bodies are disgusting (especially real ones that sweat and bleed and fall outside the narrow realm of model-type beauty) and ideally should be transcended as we leave behind the profane physical realm. For this we can thank our puritan tradition, which tells us that pleasure is sinful and we shouldn't have too much fun.

Welcome to the land of mixed messages! To be sexually desirable is essential to getting a partner and thus to happiness, but to be too sexual is a turn-off, and to be too free is dangerous and wrong. You should be great in bed (and the wilder the better!), but not a slut. You shouldn't be a prude, but not a tease, either. Just say "No." Just say "Yes." Don't say anything at all, just do it! It's okay to act wild (especially if you've got the excuse of inebriation), but to truly access your uninhibited sexual inner nature, we are told over and over again, will destroy your relationships and lead to personal ruin.

> *"Life in Lubbock, Texas taught me two things: One is that God loves you and you're going to burn in hell. The other is that sex is the most awful, filthy thing on earth and you should save it for someone you love."*
>
> **BUTCH HANCOCK**

These conflicting messages confuse people, cause enormous pain and shame, produce widespread dissatisfaction and lead to irresponsible, harmful behavior.

And some really, really bad sex.

Haunted by Our Sex-Negative Past

Historically, Western cultures have discouraged, shamed and actively banned sensuality, sexuality and the experience of ecstasy. Foundational ideas in Western belief systems such as original sin equate erotic desire with evil. Mainstream Christianity has it that the earthly body is innately bad and needs to be transcended in order to be spiritual. This is why the celibate male priest is seen as closest to the one male God and a necessary conduit to the Divine.

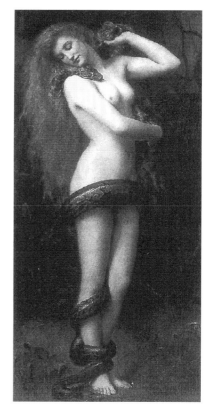

John Collier—*Lilith*

> *"Why should we take advice on sex from the pope? If he knows anything about it, he shouldn't!"*
>
> **GEORGE BERNARD SHAW**

Contemporary culture carries this baggage of thousands of years of repressed sexuality, gender inequality, aggression, fear, benightedness and oppression. It's a heavy cultural load that feeds anxiety, shame, and ignorance, and underlies sexual disempowerment. It rationalizes dominator culture and its many expressions, from slavery to the rape of the earth and all manner of violence.

Wherever You Go, There Sex Is

In our multicultural, multi-influenced milieu, we're exposed to an unprecedented barrage of sexual messages and imagery. Our pervasive (and invasive) modern media use sexuality to sell everything imaginable while dramatically limiting people's understanding of what sex is really all about. People get little information from our culture that helps them have better sex or successful intimate relationships. While a small sex-positive world culture has begun to bloom on the cultural margins, it's still difficult to find ways to understand, learn about and integrate our sexuality, or get support to heal sexual wounds.

It's a jumble out there: we live amidst a crazy mixed-up confluence of commercialized sex-fantasy images, ubiquitous sex-negative attitudes, and a budding, counter-cultural, sex-positive tide. Our muddle of a culture is at one and the same time blatantly (and unhealthily) sexual, remarkably repressed, and open to the possibility of sexual health and freedom.

What's Wrong with This (Moving) Picture?

On the silver screen, the actresses always seem to come while they're wildly, passionately and boisterously boffing. Whether it's the plumber or the man of their dreams, Prince Charming or that hot neighbor, he

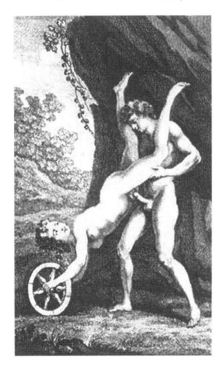

ANTOINE BOREL, c. 1780

just sticks it in, pumps away, and she comes. They often have the fabled screaming, simultaneous orgasm as the fireworks go off.

What's wrong with this picture? First and foremost, it's not real—and I mean this on two levels. First, they're acting (which everyone knows). Second, it establishes a narrative about arousal and orgasm that has little to do with reality. Most women simply don't work that way.

Our cultural portrait of what sex is all about is inaccurate in many ways. First of all, it mostly defines "real sex" as penis-in-vagina penetrative hetero-sex. To remedy this, we need to expand our definition of sex to include all the diverse ways

in which people of every sexual persuasion can experience and share erotic energy and activities. Sex doesn't even have to directly involve the generative organs! If all the "other stuff" is demoted, we are going to miss out on a wide range of erotic activity that's just as valid and important to pleasure. Kissing is sexual. Simply holding hands can be sexual! It's all "real sex" if it turns you on.

> *"Heterosexuality is not normal, it's just common."*
>
> **DOROTHY PARKER**

The most significant problem with the sex-is-fucking picture is that women and their partners often buy into the idyllic vision of cock-in-

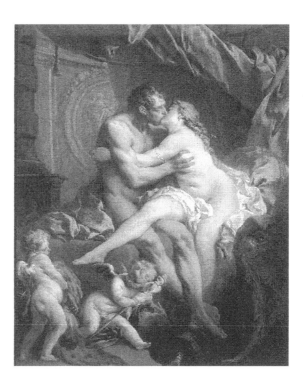

François
Boucher—
*Hercules and
Omphale*
c. 1750

pussy mediated bliss, and therefore assume that female orgasm from penetrative sex is what they should be experiencing. But that's not the reality for many women. Approximately ten percent of women have never had an orgasm at all, while over half of women don't have orgasms (screaming, simultaneous or otherwise) during intercourse. The plain truth is that for most women, fucking isn't the best way to reach orgasm.

What happens when your experience doesn't live up to the silver screen (or computer monitor) ideal? Many women conclude there's something wrong with them—something inherently, embarrassingly wrong, with little or nothing to be done about it. Who knows (they might well think), since they failed to be appropriately responsive, maybe they got gypped when the orgasmic potential was handed out!

Or perhaps a woman might blame her lover for not handing her an orgasm gift-wrapped on a silver platter. Meanwhile her confused and guilty partner is often left feeling inadequate and responsible for her failure to get off. After all, another cultural myth is that men come equipped with a set of instructions pre-printed inside their skull telling them how to turn women on.

No such manual exists, of course. Men do attend sex school, though. It's the steady stream of media images and fantasy stories that provide the template for their (and women's) erotic behavior. Unfortunately, this school imparts inaccurate and, as many men have learned to their chagrin, ineffective information. To the extent that men learn their technique from watching movies, whether it's slutty porn or fairy-tale romance, they won't have discovered what really works for women.

There is a simple explanation for this: our mainstream media model is based on masculine arousal. The irony is that since masculine and feminine sexual energy are complementary, what works for most men doesn't work for women, at least most of the time.

When sexual reality falls short of the media fantasy, people typically blame themselves (or their partners) instead of believing that our cultural model is unrealistic, limited or flawed. Instead of understanding that our sexuality includes learnable skills and we just haven't gotten good lessons yet, they feel shortchanged and stuck with a lemon of a sex life.

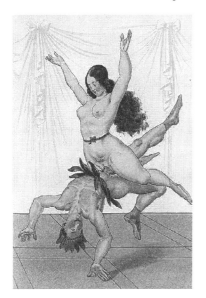

PETER FENDI—*Acrobats, c. 1830*

Sexually challenged people may go through life feeling broken, and possibly damaged beyond repair. Some repress their sexuality and channel the energy elsewhere. Others pretend they just don't care ("It's okay, I don't mind if I don't come."). Some people carry their shame in plain view while desperately trying to hide it. Others successfully keep their problems in the closet.

In addition to making many people feel as if their sexuality is somehow not up to par, our culturally-created sexual distortions have much more sinister ramifications. Some deeply disturbed people turn their sexual energy into violence, harming the innocent and often carrying the wounding into future generations. Sexual abuse, incest, assault and rape are epidemic as wounded, pathologically dysfunctional people channel their sexual energy into domination, aggression and cruelty.

Our culture consistently disempowers sexuality by manufacturing misleading images and sowing misinformation. Our media inculcate low self-esteem while holding up unachievable ideals. Our communities disrespect sexual diversity and perpetuate oppression and ignorance. We are a nation of the sexually wounded, handicapped by lack of knowledge and suppressed erotic energy that denies people their birthright—an intact and blissfully functioning sexuality.

An Embarrassment of Words

Our language for talking about sex and bodies speaks legions about our cultural shame and confusion. Embarrassment and awkwardness lurk just beneath the surface of our terminology. As I pointed out in Chapter One, our mainstream culture gives us four inadequate vocabularies—clinical language, baby talk, vague euphemisms, and so-called "dirty" words. We don't have a straightforward, comfortable language for discussing this all-important subject.

ASK DR. SCIENCE

The clinical vocabulary of the scientific world is the supposedly inoffensive, safe and superior dialect of medical professionals. Intercourse is appropriate and coitus is correct. Unfortunately, these words are anything but sexy. Can you imagine lasciviously whispering "I'd love to have intercourse with you" to a prospective partner? Can you imagine saying "Yes!" if someone asks if they can "perform cunnilingus?" Those words aren't yummy, sexy or a turn-on.

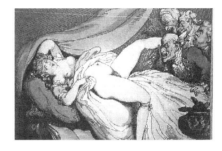

THOMAS ROWLANDSON, c. 1800

Words used by authorities and professionals have great power for good or ill. They can help us recognize our normalcy, and they can also alienate us from our bodies. There's a wide variety of normal when it comes to people's anatomy and experience. Technical words that imply otherwise can contribute to people's all-too-common feeling that they're *not* normal. For instance, the term "labia minora" means "small lips" and refers to the inner lips of a woman's vulva. Sometimes these inner lips are big, though. In fact, not infrequently they're bigger than the outer "labia majora" (or "big lips"). If a medical practitioner uses "labia minora" with a woman who has large inner lips, it's easy for her to conclude she's abnormal.

In addition to causing people to feel bad about themselves, some scientific words reflect millennia of sex-averse attitudes. When we uncover their root meanings, we find hidden negative messages. One of my least favorite words is about one of my most favorite activities. The

> *"What's the most popular pastime in America? Autoeroticism, hands down."*
>
> SCOTT ROEBEN

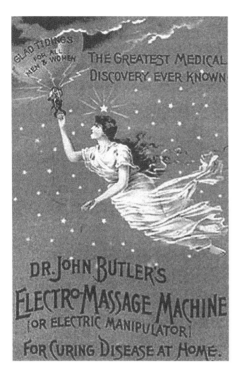

Vibrator Advertisement, c. 1900

word is "masturbation," which is derived from the Latin meaning "to pollute with your hand." That's certainly not what I'm doing when I pleasure myself! Are you?

These clinical terms have other shortcomings, too. For one thing, they can be an indirect way to stake out a power position. When an expert uses a term that a lay person may not understand, they're positioning themselves as the person in the know, and the other as an ignorant peon.

Scientific jargon can also perpetuate ignorance. Telling someone they can "get an STI (Sexually Transmitted Infection) if they perform fellatio and swallow the ejaculate" won't help if they don't know you just said they can get a sex disease from giving a blowjob and swallowing cum.

The medical community also uses its own brand of prudish euphemisms that reflect its discomfort with the subject of sex. After a pregnant fifteen-year-old who had previously denied being "sexually active" told me that she thought she couldn't get pregnant because "I'm not sexually active, I just lie there," I stopped using that phrase.

BABY, BABY, BABY

As an alternative to scientific terminology, we have the baby talk words that were used in our childhood to refer to our "private parts," words like "wee-wee," "pee-pee" and "tushy." These coy code words reflect our caregivers' discomfort with the sexual parts of our bodies. After all, there's no cute made-up word for ear or mouth.

Even if we did learn that we had a penis or vagina, many parts of our erotic equipment didn't get named at all. When you were little, did anyone tell you about your sweet little clittie?

While these words may suffice for toddlers, they don't translate well into adult sex talk, whether in the bedroom or the living room. They aren't a turn-on for most people, and they're infantilizing.

Huh? Where?

Perhaps, in your family, you didn't even have a word for your genitals. Maybe you just had vague euphemisms like "down there." Where is that, anyway? It sounds like they're talking about the 19th-century European

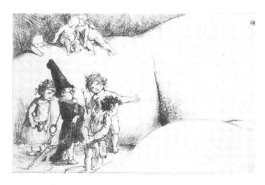

Luc Lafnet, c. 1920

concept of Africa . . . a dark, mysterious, far-away place where you'll probably never go. I guess that was the idea: if we don't name it, perhaps our darling child won't notice what they've got and will keep their exploring little hands out of their diapers.

Fuzzy, ambiguous terms like "doing it," 'hooking up" and "your thing" create a host of misunderstandings under their cloak of shame. Words like these make it difficult to describe boundaries, negotiate agreements or request specific activities.

And Your Mother!

Finally, we're left with the so-called dirty words, those bad, excitingly forbidden and racy slang terms for anatomy and sexual activities that we learned on the playground. "Dirty?" "Bad?" Excuse me? What's dirty about your amazing body parts or the arousing things you do with them? These taboo terms and prohibited phrases convey a clear message that sexuality is shameful and disgusting.

> *"There's nothing inherently dirty about sex, but if you try real hard and use your imagination you can overcome that."*
>
> **LEWIS GRIZZARD**

It's interesting to note that we use these words to insult others. Calling someone a "prick," "asshole," "cunt" or "fuck" is generally not considered a compliment. It's one more indicator of how we have culturally consigned our sexual activities to the shadows.

We need to reclaim these "dirty" and "bad" words and make them "clean" and "good."

At the end of the day, it's no surprise that our cultural lexicon makes it virtually impossible to have a straightforward, uncharged conversation about sex. What else can be expected from a society that's as confused and neurotic as ours is about the topic?

You're Not Broken

If your experience of your sexuality isn't all you wish it were, if you feel in any way inadequate or limited, ashamed of your desires or embarrassed by your deficits, please listen carefully … *it is not you who is broken*. It isn't your fault that you haven't learned the skills you need to access your pleasure, own your orgasms or heal your wounds. How many of us have been shamed for our lustful longings, secret fantasies and private acts, rather than honored for our desires and celebrated for our ability to get turned on and ecstatic! We live in a world that not only doesn't support healthy sexuality but actively undermines it, making you think there's something wrong with you or your partner.

To repeat: you're not irreparably damaged, and you didn't get cheated when they handed out sexual potential. No matter where you are sexually, you can start on the path of progress by doing one simple thing—consciously deciding to set out on a learning journey. From that point on, things will get better and better. Over time, you'll learn to access your erotic abilities, overcome your inhibitions and claim your authentic freedom.

Is Sex Sacred?

In some ancient cultures, sex was recognized as a path to the sacred Divine. It was an ecstatic practice that led to cosmic oneness and bliss and was considered proof of divine love. In these traditions, there was no distinction between mind, body, heart and spirit. All were seen as rooms in the same holy temple.

In many sex-positive cultures, sexuality was also an important part of sacred ceremony. Erotic rituals were practiced to express reverence, heal

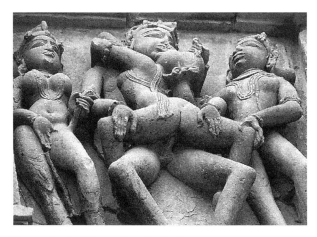

Khajuraho-Lakshana Temple, India

sickness and insure fertility. Sexual magic was used to create abundance and fruitfulness at the individual, tribal and earthly levels. The last level was the most important of all, given that Mother Earth provides everything needed to survive—our food, our tools and ultimately our very lives.

> *"Any real ecstasy is a sign you are moving in the right direction—don't let any prude tell you otherwise."*
>
> ST. TERESA OF AVILA

Tossed about as we are on the waves of our mixed-message culture, it may be difficult for us to envision sex as a joyful, loving, compassionate path involving ecstatic spiritual practice. Rituals that involve sexuality, erotic energy and ecstatic states can seem shocking and blasphemous when viewed through Western civilization's lens of profanity and shame. The reality, though, is that our sexuality has the potential to be sacred as well as intensely pleasurable. For this to happen, though, we must embrace a sex-positive, celebratory framework that honors the wonders of Eros.

Women and Sex

Throughout human history, the power accorded women and prevailing attitudes about sexuality have been inextricably intertwined. In sex-positive societies, women and the power of the feminine were honored. Indeed, women were considered especially divine as the source of life capable of growing, birthing and nourishing new beings. These cultures balanced the power of men and women, just as they honored the energies and attributes of all genders.

We do not live in a sex-positive world and can see the disastrous results all around us, including the ravaging of Mother Earth. Collectively, we can put an end to this. We can do this starting on the individual level by reconnecting our body, mind, heart and spirit with our sexuality, and by emerging from that process newly empowered.

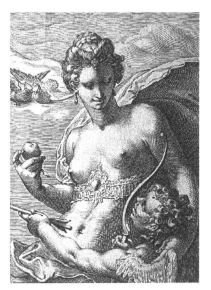

JAN PIETERSZ SAENREDAM—*Venus, c. 1590*

Orgasmic abundance is only one outcome of this. We can also access our wildness without transgressing our own or others' boundaries.

We can create sustainable intimate relationships based on being in authentic connection with our self and with others. We can learn, heal and be in alignment with our power and our purpose. We can, in short, become whole.

If we do this, if one by one we shift our consciousness in a direction that celebrates the erotic as holy, reveres both the feminine and masculine energies, and does a much better job of balancing male and female power, we will heal not only ourselves, but eventually the planet.

This is why I sometimes tell people that my mission as a teacher is to "save the planet, one orgasm at a time."

The Male Norm

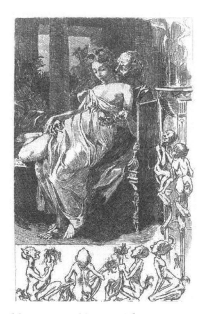

MARTIN VAN MAELE—*Thais, c. 1900*

As noted earlier, our accepted pattern of normal healthy sexuality is based on what usually works for most men. There's a tiny problem with this, of course: women aren't men. As long as women try to mimic male arousal patterns, not only will they not get what they want, but they won't discover the power of the erotic feminine. As with magnets, life exists as polarity. Our sexual model only recognizes and validates one pole. Feminine sexual energy is the other pole. It operates differently and needs to be equally understood and honored.

Most of us already understand masculine erotic energy: it's everywhere we turn, in both our porn and non-porn media. Now we also need to learn to understand the complementary energy, that of the feminine erotic.

I guarantee you: when we learn to speak both erotic energy languages and play with sexual polarity, everyone will have more fun! As they say, "When Mama's happy, everyone's happy."

The Female Mystery

The female body has always been mysterious. With their hidden genitalia, amazing ability to bleed and not die, the everyday miracle of pregnancy, the rite of passage of birthing, the ability to feed and nurture offspring,

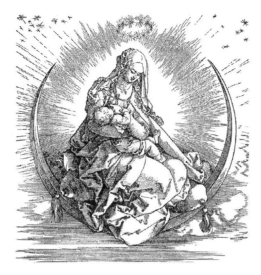

ALBRECHT DÜRER—*Life of the Virgin, 1528*

and then the time when the blood ceases to greet the monthly moon, women participate in a vast cosmic web of magic and mystery.

We live in a time of unparalleled knowledge, when many believe all mysteries have been solved, all secrets revealed. But the female genitalia still remain mysterious to both their owners and their guests. Our understandings about the feminine aspects of sexuality are limited, and often skewed by the dominant model of masculine sexuality. Our mental maps of the female body are inaccurate. Our understanding of sexuality is unbalanced towards the male perspective. It's as if we're navigating with a flawed map. No wonder it's so difficult for lots of women to get where they want to go!

What's Really Down There May Surprise You!

As an educated person, you probably think you have a pretty good understanding of both models of the standard sexual apparatus, whichever version you own or like to visit. It may surprise you to learn that our accepted cultural ideas and images of genitals are missing a lot of really good stuff.

As noted earlier, the majority of contemporary books and illustrations of female genital anatomy leave out most of the equipment responsible for arousal and orgasm. When these specialized sexual structures are omitted from our cultural images and text, they're also expunged from our mental model. The result is an ignorance that operates like a psychological chastity belt; it dramatically reduces women's sexual potential.

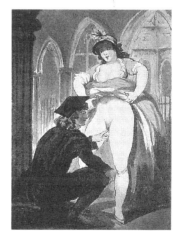

THOMAS ROWLANDSON, *c. 1800*

There is much more to women's pleasure than the clitoris (and there's more to the clitoris then meets the eye). Central to women's extraordinary, complex and elegant arousal system is what I call the erectile network, a set of structures composed of something called, you guessed it, erectile tissue. You're probably familiar with this material. It's what makes up most of the penis, giving the noble cock its much-celebrated ability to transform from a small, soft, unobtrusive organ into a stalwart and hard spire (and aren't we glad about that!).

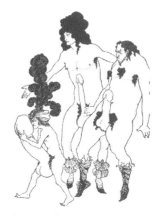

Now, here's a really important truth you probably don't know. *Women have as much of this magnificent inflatable tissue as men do!* That's right. Pound for pound, inch for inch, women have the same amount of erectile tissue as guys. So, if you thought getting turned on (or turning on your woman) was all about the tiny little hot button of the clitoris, you'll want to think again. The clit is still the lead guitar in the band … and there's also a much more extensive arousal matrix to explore and play with.

AUBREY BEARDSLEY—
*Lacedomonian
Ambassadors, c. 1890*

Although the female erectile apparatus is equivalent in size to that of the male, it's not as obvious. Most representations just show the tiny head of the clitoris, which is only the tip of the volcano. Women have an interlocking set of sexual pleasure parts, most of which are unknown or misunderstood. For women to reach their full sexual capacity, they need to discover this network of erectile circuits. When the entire system is fully activated, women can easily expand their arousal, access amazing orgasmic states and discover their deep and wondrous wildness.

This is what this book will teach you.

Playing the Whole Instrument

When we don't know what's there, we don't know how to play with it thoroughly or well, and neither do our partners. And of course we can't teach them if we don't know how to do it ourselves.

MARTIN VAN MAELE—
Presto Agitato, c. 1890

WOMEN'S ANATOMY OF AROUSAL

It's as if we've been trying to play the piano and make beautiful music, but were only aware of a quarter of the keys. With most of the keyboard missing, we can still make lovely music, but the range is quite limited. When we discover the complete network of structures and understand how the connected system works together, it's as if we now know where all the keys are (plus the foot pedals!). Once we learn how to fully play the whole instrument, we can produce a much richer and deeper range of music. Some songs that seemed well beyond our ability now become possible. We may not be able to play a Mozart sonata right away (or have a fifteen-minute orgasm), but we can see how we could get there.

Ignorance is the Opposite of Bliss

Not understanding this basic information does us all manner of harm. For starters (and most obviously), it limits our sexual pleasure, leading to dysfunction and dissatisfaction. It causes people to feel inadequate, inept or damaged. Relationships can founder on the shoals of sexual problems that stem from ignorance and deficits in basic skills.

When this lack of knowledge is coupled with the often unresolved and buried trauma of shame, sexual assault and abuse, it can compound the problems even further and produce woefully dysfunctional relationships accompanied by depression, low self-esteem, addiction and even violence.

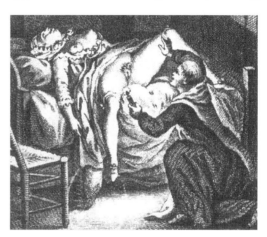

ANONYMOUS—*Candle, 18th century*

It's not just non-professionals who lack this information. This anatomy and sexuality information isn't included in standard medical training. The result: most medical practitioners don't know what's there or how it all works together. This professional ignorance produces widespread interpersonal insensitivity, epidemics of unnecessary or ill-advised medical procedures and unwonted interference with natural processes. Well-intentioned medical professionals often do more harm than good because they don't actually know what's down there.

A Brief History of Genital Amnesia and Female Sexuality

In the 21st century information age, it appears that everything about anything is available at our Internet fingertips. It seems crazy to think that we could have incomplete and inadequate cultural representations of female genitalia and sexuality, but we do. How could this have happened? How can it be that in a time of unprecedented knowledge, we could have an incomplete view of something as basic as genital anatomy?

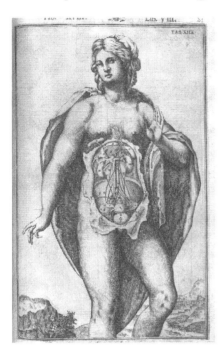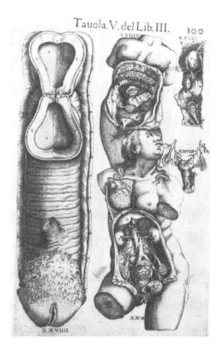

ADRIAAN VAN DE SPIEGEL and GIULIO CASSERI—From Anatomia del Corpo Humano— Female Abdominal and Pelvic Organs, and Urogenital System, c. 1600

The reasons are both simple and complex. The simplest one is that, remarkable as it may seem, the information is not generally available. Most medical, gynecological, obstetrical and midwifery textbooks as well as books for the general public on sexuality and health do not accurately depict the basic structures of the female sexual apparatus. While bits and pieces of the information are scattered throughout current and past sources, they have never been assembled and understood as a whole system.

In order to see why this is so, we need to delve a bit more deeply into the complexities of history and culture.

Prior to modern times, our ability to comprehend the human body came from observations of living beings. Then dissection came along, leading to the direct study of cadavers. Until the microscope was invented, however, we couldn't differentiate tissue at the microscopic level or understand the miniature workings of cells. Our anatomical understanding was limited to what the unmediated eye could see on (or in) a dead body.

Once information was gathered and accepted as gospel truth, that knowledge was often passed along without question to subsequent generations. Much anatomy information has come to us that way. Our contemporary model came from the last generation of anatomy books, which came from the ones before that, and so on. And much of it started off inaccurately.

It is not only our tools (or lack of them) that limit us. While the study of healing is as ancient as culture, the study of the actual structures of the body has historically been restricted. Subjective belief systems about humans and dogmatic religious traditions established what was acceptable to do and study, and what was unacceptable and profane. Whether one could actually cut up a human corpse and examine its parts was often proscribed by the religious authorities. If the body was a female one, there were additional strictures on how it could be viewed and studied.

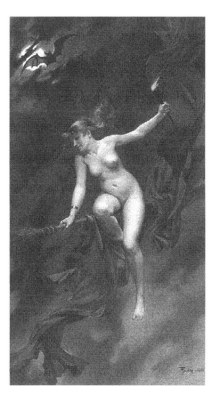

"As regards the individual nature, woman is defective and misbegotten, for the active power of the male seed tends to the production of a perfect likeness in the masculine sex; while the production of a woman comes from defect in the active power."

ST. THOMAS AQUINAS

(1225-1274)

Luis Ricardo Falero—*The Witches Sabbath, c. 1880*

Women's sexuality is a powerful force that, depending on the time and place, was revered or feared, encouraged or denied. The study of women's bodies is thus particularly fraught and tangled with ideas about how women are, what it means to be female (especially in relation to men) and beliefs about feminine sexuality.

Another reason we lack accurate information about women's pleasure systems is that images in anatomy texts have typically reflected prevailing cultural attitudes about female sexuality. As the views of women and their erotic nature shifted, the models of their genital anatomy changed with them, mirroring those cultural constructs.

In early Western culture, women were considered lusty, simple beings with a stronger sex drive then men. Early anatomy, medical and midwifery texts include female pleasure and many of the parts responsible for it.

A shift occurred with the influx of patriarchal cultures, the rise of Christianity and the ongoing struggle for political and economic power. Women were still seen as lascivious creatures, but now their carnal nature meant they were a source of evil. Females had given us original sin, were prone to seduction by the devil, and likely to drag men to hell with them.

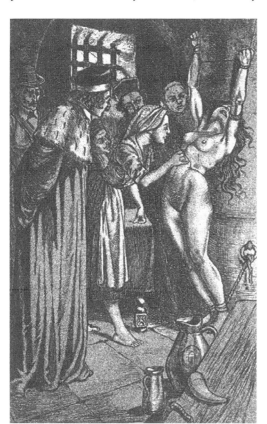

This set of beliefs brought us the madness of the Inquisition and an epidemic of femicidal witch-killings that strongly encouraged women to suppress their sexuality, to say the least.

"All witchcraft comes from carnal lust, which is in women insatiable."

Malleus Maleficarum (The Hammer of Witches)
Catholic Church's official witch hunting manual—1487

Martin van Maele—*La Sorciere, c. 1890*

Fast-forward to the Victorian era, by which time the feminine ideal had shifted away from the libidinous wench to women as pure, spiritual, asexual beings without libido or desire. Still innocent and child-like (or, shall we say, dumb), women were expected to be obedient ornaments, helpmates and mothers. They were admonished to tolerate sex as their distasteful duty to be bravely endured for husband, God and country, for the sole purpose of becoming pregnant and providing the next generation. By the 1800's, all the parts responsible for arousal and orgasm were gone from the pictures and texts in many anatomy books, while the reproductive structures remained.

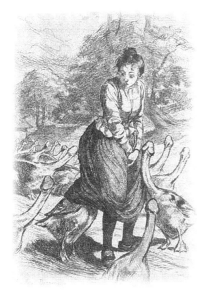

MARTIN VAN MAELE, c. 1890

"Most men are by nature rather perverted, and if given half a chance, would engage in quite a variety of the most revolting practices. These practices include, among others, performing the normal act in abnormal positions; mouthing the female body; and offering their own vile bodies to be mouthed in turn."
—Instruction and Advice for the Young Bride

RUTH SMYTHERS, 1894

As we transitioned from the Victorian era to the 20th Century, we got an important bit of female anatomy back as the clitoris was returned to anatomy books and gradually to the minds of its owners and their partners.

Cultural views of women and female sexuality have continued to progress over the last hundred years, inching ever closer to true and total gender equity and sexual empowerment. Educational barriers have been torn down, giving women access to bigger incomes and the power to better control their lives, fertility and sexuality.

In recent decades, we've made additional progress, for instance by accepting the reality of female ejaculation and the existence of the G-spot (though it's a misnomer, as we shall see). We still have a long way to go, though. We've reclaimed female libido and orgasm (yay!) and begun to rediscover the anatomy of arousal, but widespread ignorance remains about the existence and importance of the female erectile network. Hard as it may be to believe, these structures are still often unaccepted by the scientific establishment.

To sum up, then, at various times in history, all the information in this book has been known and available. We can find pieces of the erec-

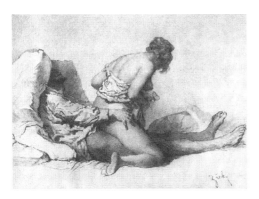

Mihaly Zichy

tile network as well as references to female orgasm (and even ejaculation) scattered in old anatomy illustrations and obscure references in medical and midwifery texts. But they didn't make it through the gauntlet of repression to our current time. In this Age of Information, critically important information is still lacking.

We are living in a culture that limits people's ability to comfortably talk about sex, celebrate their sexuality and effectively pursue their erotic potential. This leaves us with a choice. We can either let this constrain us or proactively adopt more sex-positive views and values. You will not be surprised to learn which I stand for.

This is the subject we turn to in the next chapter.

CHAPTER THREE

A Wholistic Sexuality Primer

*"When one tugs at a single thing in nature,
he finds it attached to the rest of the world."*

JOHN MUIR

The Humming in the Beehive

IF YOU'VE EVER HAD THE RARE PRIVILEGE of seeing a natural, undisturbed birth, you know that access to pleasure, intimacy and ecstasy is our birthright. Any birth is miraculous, but when you see a gently birthed baby—it's astounding. They are tiny beautiful Buddhas, quietly beaming and aglow. Watch that infant moments later, nursing ecstatically in momma's arms, and it's clear what our evolutionary template for love is.

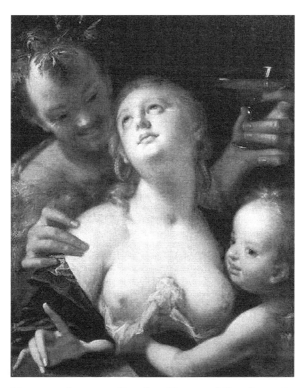

HANS VON AACHEN—*Bacchus, Venus and Cupid, c. 1595*

The word "erotic" comes from the Greek word *eros*, meaning sexual love. The poet Robert Bly said it well when he described eros as "the humming in the beehive that keeps the whole thing together." Eros is much more than the part of you that wants to have sex with other people. It's the energy that infuses the web of life from the vastness of the universe down to the tiniest microcosm. It's the force that creates life. If anything is sacred, sex is sacred.

This is the starting point of the framework I call Wholistic Sexuality, which I offer as an alternative to our variously confusing, cheapening and misleading mainstream stories about sex. Wholistic Sexuality offers an integral vision of sexual empowerment and connection that honors eros.

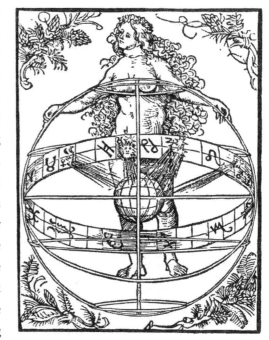

ALBRECHT DÜRER—*Nude Woman with the Zodiac*

"The mind, once expanded to the dimensions of a larger idea, never returns to its original size."

OLIVER WENDELL HOLMES

The Five Principles (Summary)

Wholistic Sexuality has five basic principles:

- Wholistic Sexuality is first and foremost about your connection with yourself.

- Sex is about all the ways we connect with everyone and everything.

- We're on a lifelong journey of learning and discovery.

- Sexual and relationship skills can and need to be learned.

- Learning depends on accurate, useful models.

Whole Sex—Macro to Micro

hy "Wholistic" Sexuality? Because it operates at every level from the macro to the micro …

WHOLE UNIVERSE: Sex is not merely an activity we do—it's an integral and inseparable aspect of all life, the manifestation of the vital energy of the universe, the world and you. In the words of the 14th century Sufi poet Hafiz, it's "the whole sweet, amorous universe in heat."

WHOLE WORLD: Sex permeates everything; its primal power affects all aspects of our world. Sex shapes our traditions, institutions, mythologies and cultures in myriad positive and negative ways. Eros fuels fertility, creativity, connection and love. It drives evolution's mix of competition and cooperation. It spawns diversity, creates beauty and generates elegant complexity. It influences all the ways humans organize themselves, including our political systems, our social systems and our spiritual traditions.

The compelling force of reproductive energy cannot be denied or annihilated, despite the effort many cultures have put into suppressing it. When the power and energy of eros is squelched, it doesn't disappear, it just becomes twisted and distorted. Then sex erupts into violence, leading to the pathological pursuit of power and driving all the vast evil that humanity has proven itself capable of.

On the other hand, when we honor the power of sexuality and channel it appropriately, we transform this earth into the garden it could be.

WHOLE CONNECTIONS: Your sexuality is about your connection to everyone and everything around you. Obviously, sex pervades your relationships with the people you choose to be sexual with, but since it's a fundamental aspect of who you are, it's also part of all your connections and interactions. Your sexuality informs your relationships with current and past intimate partners, family, friends, communities, culture, media, country and the world. It ripples out and affects everything, just as everything in the web of life affects you.

WHOLE BEING: You are a sexual being, not a sexual "doing." Sex is not just something you do—it's a fundamental and inseparable part of who you are.

Your foundational, primary sexual relationship is with yourself. This relationship is as complex, unique and individual as you are. All other relationships are influenced by your core connection with yourself.

Understanding who you are and how you operate sexually is fundamental to personal growth, self-integration and achieving your full potential.

Your Primary Relationship Is With Yourself

Wholistic Sexuality is first and foremost about your relationship with yourself. This is the most important relationship you'll ever have because it's your only truly lifelong relationship. It's where you do your most important work—your learning, growing and healing. Your sexuality is an integral, inherent and wonderful aspect of yourself.

Your sexuality is rooted in your relationship with yourself. Although our cultural model tells us that sex is about what you do with other people, those connections are actually secondary. Your true primary relationship is with yourself. All other sexual connections flow from this foundational relationship.

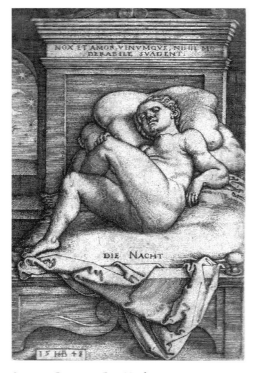

Sebald Beham—*Die Nacht, c. 1500*

"We do not go to bed in single pairs; even if we choose not to refer to them, we still drag there with us the cultural impediments of our social class, our parents' lives, our bank balances, our sexual and emotional expectations, our whole biographies—all the bits and pieces of our unique existences."

ANGELA CARTER

Your sexuality is also wholistic, encompassing your connection with all the interwoven, inseparable facets of your wondrous self and all that surrounds you. That includes your unique genetic blueprint; your physical, emotional and spiritual relationship with your body; your history and life experiences; the beliefs that you were exposed to growing up; your current beliefs and assumptions; your past and present intimate relationships; the myriad communities you're part of; our ubiquitous media; and all our many other influences. All these things together are what have formed your unique relationship with yourself and affect all your connections with the world.

For many people, many of these influences are unconscious and buried in shadow and shame. If you want to have better sex, explore your full erotic potential and have deeply healthy and sustainable intimate relationships with others, you need to begin with your relationship with

"Masturbation: the primary sexual activity of mankind. In the nineteenth century it was a disease; in the twentieth, it's a cure."

THOMAS SZASZ

yourself and bring your sexuality into the light of awareness. Only after you have done this important learning and healing work and developed a strong foundation of self-love and connection to your source can you become your own fabulous lover, and proceed from there to have your relationships with others be the healing partnerships and divine union we all yearn for.

Your sexuality, in other words, isn't only a portal to pleasure—it's also a gateway to yourself.

One thing this tells us is that you don't have to have a partner to journey to sexual wholeness. Although it's certainly fabulous to be in amorous relationships with others, it is not essential to sexual satisfaction or to leading a fulfilled life. You are always partnered with yourself.

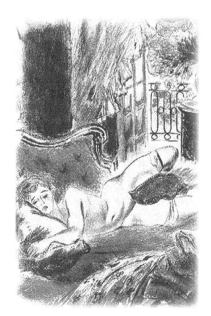

BERTHOMME ST-ANDRE, *c. 1940*

Another lesson to be gleaned from this is that, since your sexuality is centered in your relationship with yourself, it is important to give priority to how you give yourself sexual pleasure. Whatever you call it—masturbation, solo sex or self-love—it's your most important laboratory for learning and the keystone for all of your other sexual relationships. Yes, women, Wholistic Sexuality calls for you to master the art of petting your own pussy!

At the same time, please remember that your sexual relationship with yourself is about a lot more than the various ways you pleasure your juicy bits. Your self-relationship is about your connection with all the facets of your being—mind, body, heart, spirit and energy. All these connections need to be open and working for you to be in truly healthy erotic relationship with yourself. Your sexuality isn't separate—it's a healthy, natural and vital aspect of who you are. It's about the whole, not just the hole!

When you deeply and truly own your own sexuality, you gain the power to break free from the blockages of old programming, celebrate your own and your partners' pleasure and become a virtuoso of erotic expression. You can access your connection to ecstasy whenever you want to and, if you so desire, share it with others.

Once you've developed mastery of the mystery, you will have the power to create your own personal sexual revolution.

Sex Is About Connection

Sex is about connection. It's about the ways we connect with the life force, with others and with ourselves. Each of us is connected to everyone and everything around us.

At the end of the day, sexuality is about all the ways we connect. It's not something that only happens behind a locked bedroom door with select individuals. It informs all our relationships, up to and including our connection with the divine.

When you start seeing the erotic as a pathway connecting the very core of who you are with, well, *everything*, it frees you up in a way that empowers

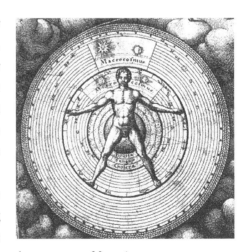

ANONYMOUS—*Manmicrocosm*

you to act in alignment with your own authentic choices. It's like rocket fuel transporting you to sexual and life autonomy:

- You can ride this erotic empowerment to choices based not on hand-me-down cultural rules, but on what will truly optimize your relationships.

- You can express your sexuality in ways that are authentic and appropriate for you, whether they be celibacy, casual dating, friends with benefits, monogamy or the increasingly popular relationship modality known as polyamory.*

- You can manage your sex life without falling prey to the confused sexual messages of our mainstream culture—for example, the message that if you're in a monogamous relationship, you're cheating in spirit if you desire other partners.

- You can conduct your relationships in a manner that honors the realities of relationship dynamics, supports the learning process of both partners and is in consummate integrity.

Despite what our culture tells us, Eros isn't something dangerous or menacing that we need to keep under wraps. Although sex has enormous power, it's a force best managed through acceptance, knowledge, integration and celebration. When we actively affirm eros, it becomes a source of pleasure, beauty, empowerment and deep and lasting connection.

A Lifelong Learning Journey

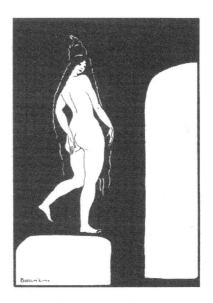

We're on a lifelong journey of learning and discovery. The universe that Shakti and Shiva launched into being is still expanding in a forever process of becoming—and, not surprisingly, so are we. We are always en route, always in transit, always learning.

Although it's not the natural way to view things, over time, many of us have come to view learning as unpleasant. This is because our formal education taught us that learning not only isn't fun—it's also

JEAN DE BOSSCHERE—*Ovid Covering Charms, 1930*

hard to do. We were taught that there's only one right answer and that making mistakes meant you were wrong and got you a lower grade.

* Polyamory: being open to or having consensual, responsible, honest relationships with more than one intimate sexual partner.

School brainwashed us into believing that knowledge comes from authorities in the forms of books and teachers, not from inside ourselves.

Real learning is a delight—an exciting adventure into undiscovered realms. It's an opportunity to develop new understanding and to achieve mastery, not in the sense of a master subduing a slave, but like a crafts-person who's become expert at their craft. The master ceramicist does not subdue the clay. Instead, by knowing its properties and using her well-honed skill, she calls forth the clay's beauty and full potential.

We are all our own master ceramicists, all here to call forth our own beauty and full potential. As much as anything, we are here to learn, to become more conscious and more skilled. Our sexuality is no exception.

The Importance of Erotic Education

Sexual and relationship skills can and need to be learned. With conscientious effort and skilled guidance, we can all become more adept sexually.

We are all on our personal journey of erotic education and have been since we were born. Like everyone else, you've already learned all sorts of things about sex, both useful and limiting. Floating in the sea of culture, you've absorbed countless ideas and beliefs. You've also probably done lots of your own empirical "hands-on" studies and explorations. However fun these experiences may have been, to fully expand your sexual

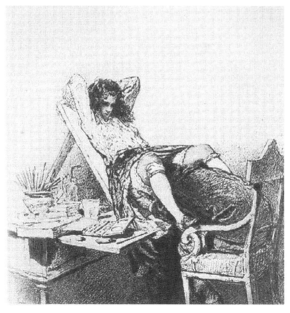

Mihaly Zichy—*Art Lesson, c. 1870*

abilities, you need to do more. You need to consciously set out to become more sexually adept.

THE FAILURE OF SEX EDUCATION

Perhaps you haven't learned to have orgasms yet, or not easily. Maybe you can have one by yourself, but not with a partner. If this is the case, that's okay. For one thing, you have lots of company, and for another, it's not surprising that you haven't acquired some or all of these more advanced abilities. After all, where would you go to learn? You certainly wouldn't get it through conventional school-based sex education! In this country, you're lucky if that teaches you how to put a condom on a banana. While that's great for safer snacking, it's not going to help you have the kind of sex you dream of.

> *"Just saying 'no' prevents teenage pregnancy the way*
> *'Have a nice day' cures chronic depression."*
>
> FAYE WATTLETON

Porn is another place people learn sexual technique, though unfortunately all you'll usually learn from that is what images and fantasies turn most men on, along with some atrocious technique.

YES, YOU CAN TEACH AN OLD DOG NEW TRICKS (OLD PUSSIES, TOO!)

We're all wired to learn. As a baby, you learned to crawl and then to walk. In a few relatively short years, you mastered the complexities of language. As an adult, you can continue to learn—to scuba-dive, play the piano or speak a foreign language. And you can also learn to have amazing orgasms.

Whatever you're studying, you won't get better overnight, not even if you spend every one of those dusk-to-dawn minutes playing with yourself or a partner. Developing a new skill has a learning curve and takes time. We learn bit by bit, accumulating knowledge and expertise, building on what we know. With diligence and commitment, though, we can get better at everything we study, including sex. Everyone can learn to expand their sexual repertoire and increase their capacity for pleasure.

That said, it's also the case that becoming more sexually adept has some special challenges. If you can't play the piano, you probably don't feel ashamed or broken. If you feel sexually inept, though, it's easy to feel inadequate. While it's perfectly understandable if you feel this way, please don't blame yourself for your lack of mastery. Where would you have learned these skills? No one thinks you're born knowing how to play an instrument, yet somehow we're supposed to know how to have great sex without the benefit of lessons or teachers.

Sex is a legitimate subject for serious (and fun!) education. It merits a place in everyone's lifelong learning curriculum.

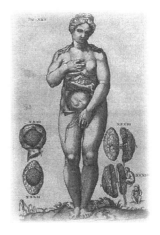

SPIEGEL *and* CASSERI—
Anatomia del Corpo Humano

The Stages of (Sexual) Learning

The process of learning goes through many stages, simplified here as three.

NOVICE: At first, you're a beginner who feels awkward, needs to think through every act and makes mistakes. When you're at this stage, it helps to remember that mistakes are normal, and being a novice is a necessary first phase. In fact, it's an opportunity to have beginner's mind and delight in newness! The cognitive scientist Marvin Minsky put it this way: it's "a chance to experience awkwardness and discover new kinds of mistakes."

Sexually speaking, if you haven't yet learned to come or if your orgasm is iffy, you're an orgasmic novice or trainee.

ADEPT: After practice, repetition and time, skills become more embodied and automatic. This is the level of the journeyman—an adept who is proficient, reliable and competent.

In sexual terms, you're at this level if you've achieved orgasmic proficiency, that is, sooner or later you can always come, using one pathway or another.

MASTER: The third level is the virtuoso—a person with true mastery of an art. An erotic virtuoso has developed extraordinary capacities such as being able to enter mega-orgasmic states or have extra-genital orgasms.

You're never done learning, even if you're a virtuoso. You're always continually exploring your art, honing your skills and discovering how far you can take them.

True and Useful Models and Frameworks

Learning depends on accurate models. To fulfill our erotic potential, we need useful maps of genital anatomy, the processes of arousal and orgasm, and more. We also need language we can use comfortably and clearly, and realistic visions of what we can achieve and how to get there.

A Great Map Gets You Where You Want to Go!

Imagine if you heard about a magical swimming hole deep in the woods. It sounds like a place you'd love to visit, where you can get naked and wet and blissful. Without a map, though, you could wander the wilds for years and never find the sweet spot you'd heard others rave about. If you don't happen to discover the path that leads to your orgasmic pond, you may wonder why everyone else seems to swim there so effortlessly. (They don't, but you wouldn't know it by all the chatter you hear about how great the swimming is there!) Maybe sometimes you do stumble into the orgasmic puddle, but at other times the path eludes you. Perhaps you decide you really want to be able to get there whenever you want to, so you buy a conventional map (maybe a sex-improvement book or a porn video) and set out to finally experience that orgasmic swimming hole for yourself. What happens when you still don't discover that magic spot? Do you conclude that there's something wrong

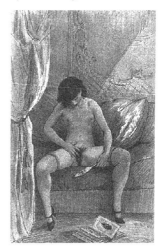

Anonymous—*An Up-to-Date Young Lady, c. 1920*

with the map . . . or with yourself? If you're like most people, you blame yourself, not suspecting for a moment that you've been misled by a false map. You may even decide that you don't really have a luscious orgasmic pond inside you.

> *"The only real voyage of discovery consists not in seeking new landscapes but in having new eyes."*
>
> **MARCEL PROUST**

As discussed earlier, to fully realize our erotic potential (and, beyond that, our potential as a culture), we need real maps that work. We especially need accurate models of women's anatomy and insightful, integral frameworks for understanding sexuality in general and feminine sexuality in particular. A good guidebook can make all the difference:

when the map actually shows you the route to the pleasure pond along with how to navigate the tricky places and the multitude of trails to get you there, your chances of getting blissfully wet are very good indeed.

To be credible and useful, these models need to prove out in the real-world laboratory of women's bodies. Genuine maps will always be congruent with actual experience, eliciting responses of "Oh, I get it! I see why that happens." When the map matches the terrain, it confirms your experience and empowers you to explore and expand. A valid map can help you find your buried treasure or, in this case, your buried pleasure!

Often, it's only in retrospect that you understand that you were lacking a map that accurately reflected your body and its abilities. When your mental picture coincides with your reality, things click into place in an extraordinary way.

Some believe our mind maps are unimportant. Sex is sex and how we visualize our bodies and the paths to pleasure doesn't matter. But it does! Our self-understanding profoundly affects how we see ourselves, how we play our sexual instrument and what we do (or don't do) with it.

In this discussion of maps and models, it's important to remember two things. First, the map is not the territory: it's an abstract portrayal, so don't confuse it with actual reality and experience. However accurate

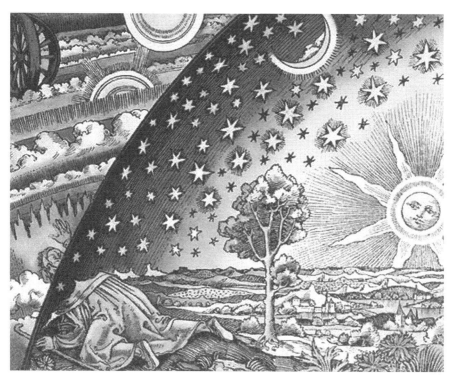

ANONYMOUS—*Edge of the Universe*

it may be, a map won't do you any good if all you do is stare at it. Unless you go out into the woods and actually follow the path it lays out, you'll never find your orgasmic swimming hole.

Second, there is never just one map of anything. The same terrain can be represented as a street map, a topographical map or a demographic one. All are true and useful in different ways. In much the same manner, different mental models can illuminate diverse facets of your being. As long as they're accurate, the more maps the better—which is a good thing, since I offer multiple models in this book.

When you journey with a valid map, it will guide you where you want to go. Inaccurate maps, by contrast, mystify, confuse and diminish us. This is why we so badly need true maps of women's anatomy of arousal, and why the need for accurate models is one of the fundamental precepts of Wholistic Sexuality. Everyone should have uninhibited access to their own wondrous wellspring of pleasure.

Whole Models of Self

Here are a few useful models of human beings and how we operate.

INTEGRAL MODEL: We are integral beings, everything is connected, and our sexuality is the inseparable and inherent life force.

ENERGY AND MATTER: We are more than examples of complex, mechanistic clockwork. We are beings that manifest out of the mysterious dance between energy and matter.

HARDWARE AND SOFTWARE: We are composed of hardware, which is what we came in with, and software, which is everything we've learned since. Sex, for humans, is both natural and learned.

INDIVISIBLE DOMAINS—MIND, BODY, HEART AND SPIRIT: We are made up of the interrelated, overlapping and inseparable domains of mind, body, heart and spirit. They exist in, and are connected by, an energy matrix.

POLARITY—THE DANCE OF LIFE: The world exists in a polarized dance of flow—like the positive and negative poles of a magnet or the magnetic fields of our planet. Night and day, inspiration and exhalation, men and women, sperm and egg, form and flow—the dualities go on and on. In the Taoist tradition, it's called yin and yang. Everyone has both polar energies and aspects within them.

WE NEED TO TALK

Words are the lens through which we see life. For this reason, language profoundly affects our mental models and thus our entire life experience. Unfortunately, as we saw in Chapter Two, our conventional language about sex reflects our cultural confusion and embarrassment about the topic.

This is not a trivial problem. How can we thoroughly explore sex unless we can communicate comfortably about every delicious, bawdy, sacred bit of it? We need to be able to talk about desire and lust. We need to discuss slippery bits and lewd fantasies. We need to feel perfectly okay with saying "making love" when we mean making love and "fucking" when we mean fucking.

"All serious daring starts from within."

Attributed to both EUDORA WELTY *and*
HARRIET BEECHER STOWE

In addition to maps that accurately reflect our real-world experience, we need a language that lets us speak about that experience easily. Words have enormous power to shape how we think, define what we're feeling and free us emotionally and intellectually. Without acceptable and yummy language, how can we hope to have a sex-positive self or culture?

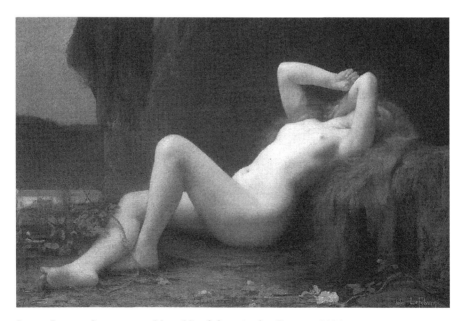

JULES-JOSEPH LEFEBVRE—*Mary Magdalene in the Cave, c. 1870*

We can all do our part in helping to create that language. I encourage you to allow your voice to come forth uninhibited by the artificial constraints of our cultural confusion about sex. Choose to be courageous and speak boldly. Set your erotic voice free!

A Toolkit of Your Own

You've already got a fabulous set of tools you can use to get turned on and orgasmic. You don't even have to strap on a tool belt (or anything else!). The basic equipment is already present in your body, mind, heart and spirit. Each of these realms has its own tools and skills, its own set of learnable abilities and techniques.

These spheres interact via the matrix of our life energy that connects and surrounds them. Electricity, biochemical messengers, emotional states, brain and heart waves and more subtle forms of spiritual energy are the strands that weave us into the inseparable and miraculous whole beings that we are.

For educational purposes, we'll treat these four realms as if they were separate. They aren't, though: they overlap and interlace.

Whether you think of these learnable techniques as tools, instruments, skills or abilities, collectively they're the key to improving your experience of both solo and partnered sex. When you train yourself to become adept at using your toolbox, you'll be able to fully access your sexual energy, get turned *all* the way on and reach amazing orgasmic heights.

Not only will you be richly rewarded in the private pleasure zone, but you'll also become a virtuoso of partner sex because we use the same tools to play with ourselves that we use to connect sexually with others. Every tool that you learn to use in your personal pleasure practice can be used during partner play to both increase your own sexual pleasure and to share erotic energy with your sweeties.

In Section Three, we'll explore these turn-on tools in more detail. For now, it suffices that, with your four-part toolkit, you've got everything you need to experience ecstasy.

Energy Matters

Einstein figured out what traditional people have known for millennia—energy and matter are two parts of one equation, the famous $E=MC^2$. Energy incarnates as the physical world we experience as solid, three-

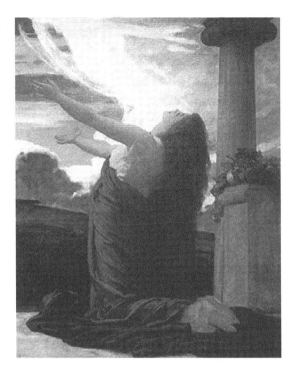

dimensional reality. Over the years, we've gradually learned to quantify energy. Early in the scientific era, we learned to measure relatively gross forms of energy such as heat. Much more recently, we've discovered how to monitor bioelectricity, recording the flickering patterns of brain waves or the pulsations of the heart's muscular rhythm.

Now scientists are beginning to figure out how to measure even more subtle forms of energy such as the powerful emotional waves that are generated by our hearts. We're gradually coming around to accept that emotional states generate energy that affects not just ourselves, but others who are nearby.

> *"The laws of gravity cannot be held
> responsible for people falling in love."*
>
> **ALBERT EINSTEIN**

We're still ambivalent about sexual energy, though. While we can measure the changes in respiration and blood pressure and so forth that accompany arousal, many are still dubious about anything more subtle and less physical. On the one hand, we take it for granted: we've all felt it, and we refer to it with words like "chemistry." On the other hand, it hasn't been officially measured ("Joe is at 73.6 erojoules and they're rising fast"), and this leaves us, in another part of ourselves, wondering if it's real or not.

In this regard, we haven't caught up with the ancient wisdom traditions of the east, who knew beyond a shadow of a doubt that not only is sexual energy real, but it's something you can work with and ride. They called it by different names—*chi, ki, prana* or *kundalini*—but it was all the same thing, the manifestation of our vital life force in the form of erotic desire. Yes—that timeless urge to merge.

These cultures developed maps and models of our energy systems that give expert guidance in how to tap into the flow. We'll be visiting some of them later in this book.

SEXUAL ENERGY: PATHWAYS TO ECSTASY

You may not think you know what sexual energy is, but I can pretty much guarantee that you've felt it. Erotic energy is the spark of attraction and the hot flowing dance of arousal. It's the rocking shuddering waves of orgasm and the wild bliss of divine union. It's what rouses males to pursue a female in musky heat and drives sperm to relentlessly seek a receptive egg. It's what sends salmon upstream, causes peacocks to flaunt, and inspires people to build palaces, fight wars, compose love songs and flash their flesh.

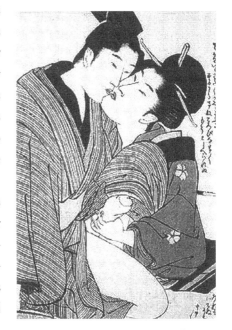

In fact, as we shall see later, it's what propels the waves of labor that push a baby out from the shelter of the womb into incarnate being. It's the vital spark that drives the reproductive imperative and the dance of existence.

You've probably experienced it many times. Do you remember

ANONYMOUS—*Exchanging Breath, 18th c. Japan*

meeting someone and having an immediate surge of interest and attraction? Can you recall a time when a lover's hands literally felt electric against your skin? When a really, really good kiss sent a wash of arousal through your body and made your knees go weak? That little buzz in your loins is your own sexual energy stirring.

Whatever you call it—passion, lust or chemistry—it's the throbbing current that you tap into in your amorous adventures, whether you're conscious of it or not. And, here's the really juicy thing about sexual energy: you can learn to amplify it and become adept at transmitting and exchanging it. You can use your toolkit to become a master of this energy.

Sexual energy is like a river of magma. Respect it, honor it, and delight in the fiery flow, but don't expect to control it. You can't. Instead, learn to open to the tide and channel its power. When you connect to the current and go with the flow, you'll find that it can enormously amplify your sexual experience.

In Section Three, we'll go into great detail about how to use your multi-faceted toolkit to hitch a ride on the *kundalini* express and ride it to orgasmic ecstasy.

CHAPTER FOUR

The Red-Hot Dance
of Yin and Yang

*"One half of the world cannot understand
the pleasures of the other."*

JANE AUSTEN

Men and Women—Different Planets or Just Different?

CAN WE LEARN TO MAKE BEAUTIFUL sexual music with partners of the opposite sex if we don't understand them? Are men and women essentially the same, or do they inhabit separate planets? I can only answer with a paradox. Men and women are erotically the same and they are also different.

Let's start with the similarities. We all operate from the same mammalian template. The basic experience of arousal and orgasm is essentially the same for everyone. As we get turned on, we breathe faster, our heart pounds and the chemical soup of arousal floods our bodies with its delicious spice. As erotic excitement builds, we tap into ancient

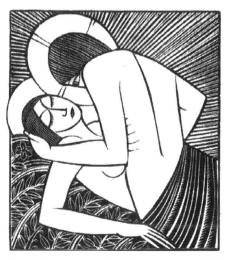

ERIC GILL—*Stay Me With Apples, c. 1900*

universal rhythms, moving unthinkingly into instantly recognizable hip-thrusting mating motions.

And yet we are deeply different too. There's a biological basis for male and female mammals (yes, humans included) to have distinct behavioral differences that reflect the imperatives of our evolutionary past. We can't escape the hormones and structures that developed for the survival of our species. Women are designed to grow, birth and nurse babies, and men are not. We live with the hardware ramifications of our ancient mating and child-rearing requirements.

To add to the complexity, we also have cultural programming that defines the genders, assigning differing attributes to each. Social concepts of gender, including what is appropriate for each and even how many there are, are varied and diverse.

There is also enormous individual variability. Some women are very feminine and others quite masculine, with every possible combination in between. Men have just as much variability. Add to that the biological, genetic and congenital variations on the male-female theme and we get quite a mosaic of possibilities.

Still, we can make some generalizations that hold true more often than not. For example, what turns each of us on differs, but often bifurcates along gender lines. Just look at who buys romance novels and who buys Playboy! As a class, men and women tend to be quite dissimilar.

"Seems to me the basic conflict between men and women, sexually, is that men are like firemen. To men, sex is an emergency, and no matter what we're doing we can be ready in two minutes. Women, on the other hand, are like fire. They're very exciting, but the conditions have to be exactly right for it to occur."

JERRY SEINFELD

How are we to make sense of this complexity? Can we understand our similarities and differences in a way that will enable us to find commonality while appreciating individuality, diversity and our unique and authentic selves? Can we get past our confusion, appreciate our differences and deeply and truly connect? Can Martians visit Venus, and vice-versa? The answer is an emphatic yes.

To do so, however, we must focus on *energy*, not *anatomy or gender*. There is masculine energy and there is feminine energy, and we all have them both in varying measure, whether we identify as a man or a woman or somewhere in between.

A Cosmic Tango

Although we tend to think of masculine and feminine energies as opposites, they're not—they're *complementary*. They create polarity, a scientific word for attraction that can be equally applied to the positive and negative poles of two magnets, the poles of the earth and the powerful pull of desire.

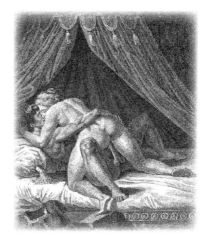

Agostino Carracci—
Mars and Venus, c. 1580

It's the interplay of these energies that creates attraction, stimulates mating behavior and leads to sizzling sex. And you know what? You don't have to be heterosexual for this fabulousness to happen. The energy is still complementary when men partner with men, or women with women, since it's the polarity, not the particular genitals, that creates the attraction.

Whether you're a man or a woman, you have both masculine and feminine aspects inside yourself. Tough guys sometimes yearn for *amour*. Dreamy romantics sometimes like to check out sexy flesh.

Neither of these forces is good or bad, better or worse. Nor is one type of energy superior to the other. The power of the feminine is equal but not identical to that of the masculine (an important point that patriarchal types tend to dispute).

Masculine and feminine energy interact dynamically to mitigate and strengthen each other in homeostatic interplay, together creating a living, integral, whole system.

There's a name for this system: life. Male and female energy in their cosmic dance are the source of, that's right, *everything*.

The Tao of Sex

To have more erotic fun, deepen intimacy, and meet your own and your partners' deepest yearnings, you need to understand the dynamics of these complementary energies. It's a model that can get us beyond cultural stereotyping about what it means (or should mean) to be a man or woman to being more in touch with our authentic nature.

Doing this doesn't require us to get ahead of the curve. Instead, we need to get *behind* it. Ancient cultures built elegant, sophisticated philosophies around the concept of sexual energy. In the Taoist teachings in particular, we find a very useful tool for understanding gender differences.

Let's take a closer look at the ancient Taoist wisdom of yin and yang.

Understanding Yin and Yang

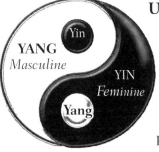

There is light and dark, day and night, sun and moon … none is right or wrong; neither is better or worse. Without light, all would be formless darkness. The night allows you to appreciate the glory of flame; the day makes possible the beauty of shade. Both aspects are beautiful and needed.

The root meaning of the words yin and yang refers to the dark and light sides of the mountain. The ancient Taoists understood that the universe is composed of two fundamental forces that move in harmony. There is day and night, inhalation and exhalation, energy and matter. The Taoists also understood that we always need both, that life can be seen as a dance of polarity between these complementary energies.

Our world and everything in it is composed of these polarities. Together, yang and yin energy form a flowing, harmonic whole.

BEING BOTH

Let's look deeper into the two basic energetic patterns. Yang is the steady, hot, fiery force associated with masculine energy and the sun. Yin is the fluctuating, cool, watery power connected with feminine energy and the moon.

Masculine and feminine, yin and yang, estrogen and testosterone—we all have both, in varying amounts and in our own unique equation. Even macho men and girly girls aren't 100% one or the other. Everyone has at least a bit of each within them.

CORE AND COMPLEMENT

Taoist sexual teachings tell us that most of us have one pole that's stronger and more central, while the other forms a weaker secondary force. While everyone has both yin and yang qualities, for most people their primary energy creates their core nature, comprised of their stronger characteristics, traits and tendencies. Our secondary energy complements the core force, balancing and leavening its power.

Most women's core energy is yin, while for most men, yang is central. As we've seen, though, individual mileage does vary. There are some women whose core is yang, while some men are predominately yin. A small number of people are evenly balanced between the two energies and can go either way. An even smaller percentage of folks seem to be utterly neutral and are completely asexual (and probably not reading this book!). For most people, however, one force will be more central and compelling than the other.

YIN FLOW

Yin, which as we have seen is typically associated with feminine energy, is like cool water, slowly flowing and yielding. The yoni typifies yin in its ability to open and close. When yin feels secure,

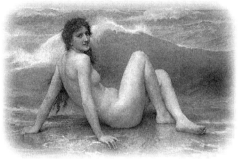

ADOLPHE-WILLIAM BOUGUEREAU—*The Wave*

it relaxes open, dilates and receives what is offered. Yin is flower-like—it blooms. It surrenders to opening, but only when it feels safe to do so.

Yin energy is lunar. Women are much more changeable then men due to the many shifts in hormones and energy of their fertility cycle, as well as pregnancy, birth, breast-feeding and menopause. Female arousal and sexual energy reflect the fluctuations of the moon, encompassing a multitude of shifts and changes. Indeed, women's fertility cycles used to be tuned to the moon's cycle before the influence of modern life (particularly artificial light) changed that. Yin energy flows and fluxes, waxes and wanes in a process of constant transformation.

Yin begins outside our physical self, past the perimeters of the body, in the space between people: it is held by relationship, by connection. Yin is process-oriented, enjoying the journey and not particularly focused on the goal. Yin energy proceeds from the edges, gradually moving inward and flowing downward toward the sex center. For sexual arousal to happen (and childbearing, too), yin needs time to accumulate and coalesce.

Since yin energy flow must pass through all the other energy centers before it reaches the genitals, it's subject to energy blockages, inhibitions and distractions. One place where arousal often gets stymied is the safety center, the energy vortex just below the genitals. A woman won't get turned on if her arousal impulse is stifled before it reaches her crotch.

Yin energy needs to pass through the heart center before it descends lower. This explains why, generally speaking, women find it harder than men to separate sex from love. Most women need to feel connected and safe before they can open up and receive in an active and conscious way.

It's no coincidence that pussies and hearts are similar in important ways. Neither can be forced to open, only invited and encouraged to do so. You can't force yourself to fall in love, and you can't make your body open, either.

This isn't to suggest that the heart and yoni can't be influenced by their yin-centered owners. You can hold an intention to keep the heart open and to open sexually, too. You can choose to be open to both love and lust. Intention and conscious choice make these things likelier to happen, but they hold no guarantees. At the end of the day, the heart makes its own decisions and the yoni does, too.

Yin qualities include a great ability to multitask, to see the big picture and have wide and diffuse perception. These are great qualities if you're making business phone calls while doing laundry and planning dinner. They're not so great in the bedroom, though. Yin is susceptible to diversion and interruption, which is why women are more apt to become distracted during sex and stray from the path of sexual arousal.

Finally, yin energy helps explain why most women take longer to become aroused than men when engaged in partnered sex play. As we've seen, yin needs to feel safe and connected in order to get really turned on. Her energy needs to flow freely through all of her. She needs protection from distractions that might get her busy brain buzzing. She needs time since it takes longer to boil a pot of yin water than to get a yang blaze roaring.

"Sexual pleasure in woman is a kind of magic spell; it demands complete abandon."

SIMONE DE BEAUVOIR

This can create a challenge for yang-centered people. They need to learn to keep their fire burning long enough to bring yin's water to a raging boil.

The good news here is that once you get the yin temperature up, the water can stay hot for a very long time. It can also be brought to a boil again quickly. Not only that, but the more frequently you bring her erotic energy to a boil, the easier it will be to get her hot tomorrow. Unfortunately, if that yin water hasn't gotten any heat lately, it has a tendency to get icy and may even freeze.*

Once yin has relaxed and received, she has a special and most

---

* It's not a coincidence that women who have arousal and orgasm dysfunction used to be called frigid. The reality, though, is that they don't feel cold so much as unsafe due to experiences such as sexual abuse or the ministrations of well-meaning but unskilled lovers.

Timing, Teasing and Tantalizing

You'll get a much more enthusiastic response to your sensual and sexual ministrations if you remember to make sure that she's already moderately aroused before you touch her tender bits. Tease, tantalize, hover and graze her hot spots before you zero in for concentrated attention. Start from the edges and work your way towards the center. Circle your target instead of instantly aiming for the bulls-eye. The challenge is to inspire her to open up and expand out towards you, inviting and drawing you in. When you dive into her crevices too soon, she'll contract, freeze and close up. In fact anytime you feel her contracting or withdrawing, it means you've probably moved in too soon. It's always better to proceed more slowly to your target than to go too fast!

This is the most common complaint about men, so prove you're not one of "them" by taking your time to awaken her whole body, arouse her desire and let her erotic energy accumulate in her sex center before you plant yourself there.

miraculous ability—the magical power of transformation. The magic of yin lies in this: when it receives a gift, it can perform alchemy. This is most clearly demonstrated in the miraculous cauldron of conception, pregnancy and birth. Yin receives seed, mixes it magically with her egg and then over the course of ten moons transforms that fertilized cell into a baby, birthing something totally new into the world.

The yoni and the womb embody yin's energetic ability to alchemically create the gold of new life. Whether it's a tiny new being, a work of art or a revolutionary vision, yin magic is at work when we receive inspiration, cook it inside and birth our new creation into the world. When yin is held safely, opened lovingly and receives your offering, you can be sure that she'll shower abundance back out, whether upon her lover or as a gift to the greater world.

YANG FIRE

Yang energy is fiery, fast and focused. It's outgoing, active and assertive. It initiates and directs. Yang is associated with masculine attributes and qualities and is most often the core energy of men. The stalwart erect phallus is the essence of yang. The wang is yang and loves to bang. It moves in and out, penetrating and withdrawing. Yang seeks to enter, to insert and get to the center. Impatient with delay, it wants to get where it's going by the most direct route possible.

Yang is penetrating—both in the sense of entering (and sometimes barging in), and also discerning, comprehending and getting to the bottom of things. Yang energy fuels the masculine chase, the hunt, the pursuit of desires. Folks with core yang energy tightly focus, aim for the target, fight off the competition and drive toward the goal.

"Anybody who believes that the way to a man's heart is through his stomach flunked geography."

ROBERT BYRNE

Male arousal and yang sexual energy can be thought of as solar—tuned to the simple repeating rhythm of the daily circadian cycle. While changes do occur over time, male life transitions are usually quite gradual. Yang energy is steady and consistent.

Yang likes surfaces, especially things that stick out, like nipples and cocks and all things that rise and point and poke. Yang arousal is easily stimulated by the visual: it loves to look at all the juicy potential targets out there.

Yang energy originates in the genitals. For many if not most yang men, you could simply dive in and initiate sex play with direct genital stimulation, and they'd be happy as a clam. (Probably considerably happier, since clams don't have genitals.)

"The common thread that binds nearly all animal species seems to be that males are willing to abandon all sense and decorum, even to risk their lives, in the frantic quest for sex."

RANDY THORNHILL *and* CRAIG T. PALMER

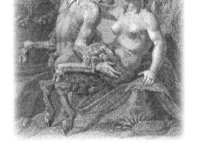

Based on AGOSTINO CARRACCI— *Culte de Priape, c. 1580*

Once fired up, that hot yang sexual energy can stay right there in the pelvis and explode in a genital ejaculation without having to pass through any of the other energy centers. Or—and we're talking about more mature yang here—that same yang energy can be trained and directed to move upwards and outwards, becoming deeper, wider and more inclusive.

A lot of male sexual behavior can be explained by this combination: the quick heat of their own arousal, its genital location, and our cultural support for unbalanced yang sexuality (about which more below). This is why more men than women are apt to be totally okay with sex that's a genitals-only connection. It also helps us understand why untutored, excessively yang lovers want to dive right into genitally-focused sex with a "How soon can I put it in?" attitude.*

Core Yin and Yang

CORE YIN	CORE YANG
• Starts at the edges	• Starts in the center
• Feminine	• Masculine
• Vagina	• Penis
• Cool	• Hot
• Watery	• Fiery
• Slow	• Fast
• Inward	• Outgoing
• Wide focus	• Tight focus
• Process-Oriented	• Goal-Directed
• Passive	• Active
• Reticent	• Assertive
• Receptive	• Penetrative
• Whole body focus	• Genital focus
• Slave	• Master
• Sustains	• Initiates
• Subtle	• Direct
• Lunar	• Solar
• Fluctuating	• Steady
• Movement	• Stillness
• Cooperative	• Competitive

THE DEEPER DANCE OF YIN AND YANG

The Taoists' insight into the nature of things goes deeper than the single, simple contrast between yin and yang, profound though that is. Within each energy, there is also the seed of its opposite. Yin contains yang and yang contains yin. Both forces are always present, each held within the other, in a grand dance of cosmic balance.

---

* Porn doesn't help, either. It invariably cuts to the genital chase without displaying any non-genital foreplay. This is because men are likely to find it boring, even though the female performers require it to get aroused enough for the main event.

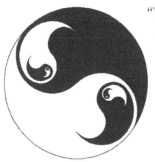

"There is a pair of opposites in all things, and in each there exists the spirit of the opposite: in man the quality of woman, in woman the spirit of man, in the sun the form of the moon, in the moon the light of the sun. The closer one approaches reality, the nearer one arrives at unity."

SHERI WINSTON—
Yin Yang Seeds Within

HAZRAT INAYAT KHAN

The Yin and Yang of the Feminine. The female reproductive organs provide a clear example of how yin contains yang. Basic feminine energy is exemplified by the vagina and womb, which are eminently capable of opening, receiving and nurturing. Yet nothing is so powerful as the womb when it's pushing new life out into the world. This is the "yang feminine"—the spontaneous and unstoppable power of birthing, the great cosmic force that impels creation out.

The Yin and Yang of the Masculine. Just as yin has a masculine aspect, yang has a feminine aspect. Again, let's go to the genitals: the yang masculine is exemplified by the stalwart phallus. This is the focused, goal-oriented, active, thrusting force. In contrast to this expanding, penetrating energy, there's the masculine's yin aspect, which is exemplified by the tender testicles. The testes have the quality of husbanding—holding the abundant seeds of the future, patiently allowing them to ripen in their safe container.

Yin Masculine and Yang Feminine

YIN MASCULINE	YANG FEMININE
• Testicles	• Uterus
• Hold	• Birth
• Husbanding	• Mothering
• Stewardship	• Parturient
• Containment	• Releasing, Ejecting
• Seeds	• New Life

An Unbalancing Act

In our culture, it's often the case that we've over-developed one pole while the other is ignored, disowned or disdained. If this is your situation, your imbalance will be reflected in your life and your relationships. Some people may need to learn to cultivate a weak core, while others will need to strengthen a fragile complement.

UN-COMPLEMENTED CORE

One major part of our dysfunctional cultural model of gender, of what it means to be a "real man" or a "real woman," is due to a false ideal of core energy without its complement. The secondary energy is needed to moderate and mitigate the primary one. Without our complementary energy to regulate our core power, we have problems.

UNBOUNDED YIN—THE DOORMAT SYNDROME

When core yin energy is unbalanced by yang, the result is weakness, passivity and submission. A person with uncomplemented yin energy is the doormat anyone can walk on. People who stay in abusive intimate relationships suffer from unleavened yin. They open when love is present and close when violence is perpetrated upon them. Without the countering effects of healthy yang, they lack an inner guardian to protect them. Instead, they just take it. Yang's directionality could help them leave, but they don't have it.

UNMITIGATED YANG—INDIVIDUAL AND CULTURAL VIOLENCE

Yang energy unleavened by yin penetrates without regard for the recipient's desires. It is the archetypal rapist, a term I use here to describe anyone who perpetrates violence for the sake of wielding power over others.

Most cultures on the planet today are tilted unhealthily toward the yang. They value conquest and dominance, and focus on short-term gain and goals without regard for means. This imbalance is at the

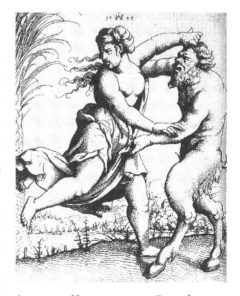

AUGUSTIN HIRSCHVOGEL—*Struggle between a Satyr and a Woman, c. 1530*

heart of much of the confusion, violence and unhappiness that character-
izes contemporary culture. Imbalanced yang energy fuels every manner
of dysfunction, from the young man who thinks there's something wrong
with him because he doesn't mirror the pathologically yang norm to the
date rapist who doesn't accept a "No." It also operates at multiple levels,
including the out-of-control lynch mob and every form of war, corporate violence and systematic aggression.

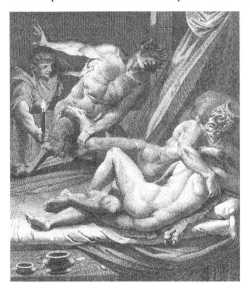

Based on AGOSTINO CARRACCI—*Pandora c. 1580, printed 1798 by Jacque Joseph Coiny*

Unblocked, the life force flows into sexual life energy, creativity, love and service. Suppressed and distorted, it takes the form of internally-directed aggression such as depression or self-sabotage, or external aggression such as rape, conquest and institutionalized violence.

Our world is being savaged by unmitigated yang. But if we can find our way to equally valuing the masculine and the feminine, we'll find the balanced path we and our world so badly need. Honoring both yin and yang is immensely important not only for each of us personally, or just to create harmonious intimate relationships, but for the well-being of the wider world.

A SUPPRESSED CENTER

Another familiar problem occurs when we act primarily out of our secondary energy in order to succeed in the world or our personal relationships, at the expense of ignoring or downplaying our core energy. A core yin woman who works as a high-powered executive may have ignored her core energy while over-emphasizing her secondary power to succeed in what is both literally and figuratively a man's world. A core yang man may have been guided by the norms of his sub-culture to pursue love (and sex) by being a sensitive New Age guy. This sort of man is great at yin skills such as listening and nurturing, but it comes at the price of his yang power, and because most (yin) women hunger for that yang energy, it also often comes, to his massive disappointment, at the cost of his getting laid.

The Beauty of Balance

Ideally, both our core and our complementary powers will be well-developed (though not necessarily *equally* developed) and in healthy balance, thereby completing each other.

HOT YANG LEAVENED BY SWEET YIN

When someone (usually but not always a man) has yang energy as his core power, he seeks to penetrate with his tight focus and nail the target. He lusts to do, to initiate, to enter and achieve.

If he also has well-developed secondary yin, he'll be interested in putting out only what another wishes to receive, in penetrating only what is offered to him. When

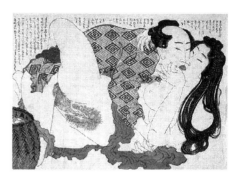

KATSUSHIKA HOKUSAI—*Shunga, c. 1800*

healthy central yang energy is complemented and leavened by yin, he will practice the all-important skills of *appropriate and attuned giving*. He'll proffer his gifts to the world in loving service. He'll be the master lover, using directionality and focus to give his partner what she most wants to get, precisely how and when she wants it. Yum!

Yang fire mellowed and mitigated by yin results in penetrating your partner with love. Yang evolved and balanced is about service. It is the archetypal energy of the Lover serving his Beloved. It is also the energy of the Warrior who protects all that is fragile and precious from those who would harm it.

Please remember that although my focus is on yang energy, this is not about people with penises—it is a gender-neutral description. All of us, women too, need an Inner Lover, an aspect of ourselves that wants nothing more than to gift the ones we love with bliss. We also all need an Inner Warrior who guards us and will give everything, including their life, in that service. Yang healthily complemented by yin is as much the fierce tigress protecting her kits as it is the knight in shining armor.

YIELDING YIN BOUNDED BY VIGOROUS YANG

Yin energy is the power of reception. Yin has the essential quality of opening and yielding or of being able to close, tightly furled in protection.

When yin is balanced, supported, and fortified by well-developed yang, a woman (or anyone with core yin energy) is discerning in her choices of who and what she'll receive. She'll practice *active reception*—consciously deciding if and when to open, then actively and enthusiastically taking in what she desires.

Yin must feel secure and protected in order to allow herself to open. Active reception means that a woman trusts in herself and her ability to choose partners who honor her boundaries and will be appropriate and attuned lovers. When yin feels safe, she can allow the ultimate surrender, opening more than she ever imagined possible, abandoning herself and succumbing to complete yielding. This is when yin energy magic happens and what has been received undergoes mystical transformation and is showered back out in blessed abundance. Yin that is forced open or pressured to yield unwillingly cannot give that gift.

The Pussies' and Puppies' School of Love

To help you better understand how yin and yang energy play out in men and women, I offer one more metaphor—the pussies and puppies paradigm. You play differently with the two kinds of animal and have differing expectations of each. You don't expect your yin kitty to fetch or your yang puppy to purr! Welcome to your personal pet (or is it petting?) store!

PLEASING THE PUSSY

Let's start with pussies. Most cats demonstrate many of the qualities we associate with yin energy. Imagine that you wish to befriend a new kitty. Since you're the one who's seeking to pet the pussy, you're being the yang one here. You could just rush up and grab the cat, flip her over and start to rub her belly. If you did this, you probably wouldn't get too far before she scratched you, hissed and took off, assiduously avoiding your grabby paws in the future. Alternatively, you could try to

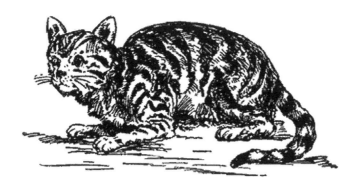

EDWARD LEAR—*Pussycat*

dominate her with your strength—maybe subdue her and tie her up, though it's hard to imagine doing it without incurring some serious damage—but that wouldn't get you the puddle of purring pussy you want either, would it? With our feline friends, force and impatient pursuit don't cut it.

Of course that's not how you approach her! Instead, you mediate your yang desire with yin skills—you woo her in an attuned and appropriate way. First, you get her attention and make eye contact. You approach slowly, gauging her response. After all, some kitties are friendlier, while others are quite skittish. Next you offer your hand for her to sniff, quietly reassuring her about your intentions. When you see that she's okay with your approach to her, only then do you begin to touch her. You probably start off with broad firm stokes along her back, relaxing her, demonstrating your attunement and the pleasure you can give her.

As she learns to trust you, Ms. Yin Kitty opens and relaxes. Maybe she rubs her face against your hand, asking for more, so you start to stroke the more sensitive areas of her neck and throat. If you take your time, focus your attention on her and read her messages correctly, eventually you'll have the lapful of purring pussy you were hoping for. The more she comes to know and trust you, the sooner she'll relax and grant you full access, surrendering to you and her own pleasure.

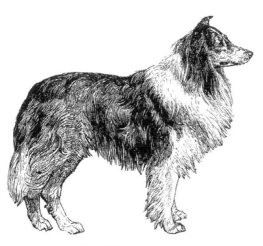

ANONYMOUS—*Good Dog*

PUPPY POWER

Dogs are active, full of energy, and always up for a romp. Puppies are eager and animated—they're just so much fun to play with! Enthusiastic, hot-blooded, ardent yang is embodied in our loyal friend, the canine.

Dog energy is extroverted and outgoing. When you meet a new dog, it doesn't take long before he greets you with a friendly inquisitive sniff. Usually, pretty much anyone can pet him. It won't take long before Fido is lolling at your feet, offering his belly and begging to be rubbed. ("Woof … please rub it … please rub it, please … please, please rub it!")

Dogs are focused and goal-directed. When you're playing fetch with a dog, they're totally zeroed in on the ball, determined to track and fetch it back for you. When they're pursuing a hot scent, they're on the trail and nothing will deter them till they find what they're seeking.

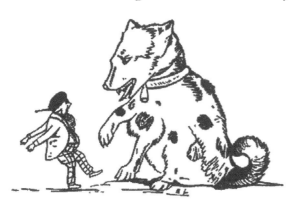

EDWARD LEAR—*Bad Dog*

If well-trained, the dog will be undistracted by other goodies along the way, though a poorly disciplined pup may run off after every sniff of a tasty morsel.

An undisciplined dog is the epitome of poorly balanced yang energy. He jumps up and knocks you over with his untutored desire to connect. He sticks his nose in your crotch, paws at you with clumsy enthusiasm and just won't leave you alone. He might even hump your leg! Unrestrained yang energy is a sixteen-year-old boy with a hard-on or a puppy who wants to go for a walk. Either way, they impatiently poke and prod. "Now?" they ask imploringly. "Now? Can we do it now? No? Well, how about now? Now?"

Contrast this with a mature dog (or lover) who waits patiently and doesn't strain at the leash. Whether he's a pooch or a sex partner, his doggy yang energy is disciplined and appropriate. Well-trained dogs don't bowl you over with their uncontrolled lust or bug you with their relentless desire to play hide the salami.

"A gentleman is a patient wolf."

HENRIETTA TIARKS

Dogs are renowned for their loyalty to the ones they love. The dog is a top-notch guardian, protective of his family. He is a warrior bravely fighting off danger and rescuing those in need. Dogs love to serve and are happiest when they have a job to do. Whether he's fetching a ball or herding sheep, he's joyfully putting himself to use—serving with enthusiasm, energy and focus, and wanting only to be loved in return.

This is yang energy at its finest. When yang is beautifully leavened by yin, you don't just have a "good dog," you have a great dog! And a great lover, too.

Your Personal Polarity

As you've been reading these pages, you've probably been asking yourself what your mix of yin and yang is. It's an important and useful question. The more you know yourself in this regard, the better you'll be able to understand your sexual choices and behavior, and the sort of work you need to do to become more whole.

The first thing to identify is your natural balance relative to your core and complementary energies.

Your sexual energy template is your unique pattern. It's part of your hardwiring, and although it may be partly due to deep early programming, it doesn't appear to be amenable to change. It may take some time for you to discover your true nature in this regard, particularly if you don't fit one of the more common gender stereotypes.

I encourage you to honor your yin and yang mix, whatever it may be. No energetic pattern is right or wrong. Our uniqueness is a blessing, not a liability. We are what we are, threads in the marvelously diverse tapestry of life.

To discover your default settings, ask yourself some simple questions. Are you like most people, with one polarity stronger and more central? Or are you evenly balanced, with equal parts yin and yang? If you do have a dominant core energy, is it yin or yang? What is your natural way of being most of the time? Remember, we all have both energies, so the question isn't if you're ever yin or yang, it's which one is active more of the time.

Next, give thought to how evenly divided or disproportionate your primary and secondary energies are. The more difficult it is to answer this question definitively, the closer you probably are to fifty-fifty.

Here are more questions you might ask yourself. Do I prefer to offer or pursue? Would I rather be held or do the holding? Do I prefer to initiate or entice? Do I feel more at home in a dominant or submissive role? Am I the bitch in heat sending out my hot scented invitation, or am I the wild alpha wolf taking my willing prey?

Yin radiates attraction and yang goes after it. If in your deepest desires and fantasies, you want to surrender in openness, you are core yin.

If your utmost desire is to open, enter and fill your lover, to penetrate and suffuse her, to melt her into oblivion, your core is yang.

Whole and Balanced

No, I'm not talking about Fox News. I'm talking about you, or rather the highly evolved self you are or can be. Now that you've got a better sense of your yin-yang mix, the next step is to get more clear on the extent to which you've fully developed both polarities. Ask yourself, do I have full access to each? Have I cultivated both my receptive yin and my doing yang? Some people have one of these areas down pat, while the other feels like scary foreign territory. Note your strengths, gifts and passions. Look at what comes easily to you and then note your challenges, weaknesses and hidden shames. Do you tend to be impatient? Then perhaps you need to develop your yin aspect. Do you have trouble asserting yourself? You may need to work on your yang.

Nowhere is your energetic nature more transparent than in the intimate sexual arena. You'll usually be attracted to people whose pattern fits with yours like two interlocking puzzle pieces. Not only will your partner's dynamic be the opposite of yours, but it will often reflect your undeveloped aspects. If your yin is immature, for instance, it's their yang that is likely to be weak.

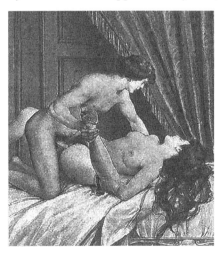

EDOUARD-HENRI AVRIL—*Polly Philips and the Young Italian*

The more we develop a healthy inner balance, the likelier we are to be drawn to partners who are healthier, too. Whole and balanced attracts whole and balanced.

To reach our full potential, we need to nurture both our dominant and subordinate aspects and the ability to move between them. When you are the master (or mistress) of your polarity, you can dance fluidly between your two energies. You can access your full range of skills and abilities, appropriately summoning whichever are needed.

LEARNING TO DANCE

We can all learn to become proficient in accessing both yin and yang energies, in getting our blaze going and boiling our water. Our first step, however, must always be to look inside and see where we need to develop. We need, in other words, to learn to polish both our core and complementary qualities. When we learn to tap deeply into our core energy while dancing with our complementary one, we unleash our full sexual potential.

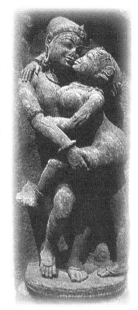

Core yin folk (usually women) can learn how to honor their yin-ness and do what's required to feel connected and fully empowered, opening all their energy centers so their energy doesn't get blocked. They can also learn to access their own yang energy, focusing fiery heat as necessary to bring their water to a rapid boil.

Core yang people (usually men) can learn how to use their focus to concentrate not on getting as quickly as possible to the promised land, but on how much fire they can bring to the journey, and how deeply they can feed their partner's arousal. They can be yang by bringing their active lust and intention to create delight and

Ancient Temple Carving, India

connection, and yin by consciously slowing down, opening and receiving, and moving their arousal from their genitals to their whole body.

This process doesn't only benefit us as individuals. As we gain insight into ourselves, we can take what we've discovered and use it to support our partners in their parallel learning journey.

The Wisdom of True Sexual Maturity

It takes a long time for human animals to become sexually mature, by which I mean something very different from *reproductive* maturity: we're able to reproduce long before we're ready for the responsibilities of parenting or partnering. It takes most people decades to reach their full sexual potential. Although our culture equates ripe sexuality with youth, true sexual maturity is often accompanied by soft bellies, gray hair and wrinkles.

"We have it in us to be splendid."

MAYA ANGELOU

As people age, they often become more adept at accessing different aspects of themselves, including their complementary energy. The best lovers are sages— mature people who are able to act in alignment with their authentic self and to be in ongoing, conscious connection with others. You've reached true sexual maturity when you can appropriately use the full spectrum of your core and complementary powers, whether that be in the sacred sex temple, the bedroom or the boardroom.

How to Slow Down and Come All Over

The inherent variability of female sexuality can be confusing to people who like to follow formulas, push buttons and get the same results every time. The yang fire is quick to ignite and, if not husbanded carefully, also quick to burn out, leading to premature extinguishing, which is something no man (or woman) wants. If you're yang, you need to keep your fire burning long enough to boil her water (and, ideally, keep it boiling for a very long time). The mature and attuned yang lover enjoys the twists and turns of the journey, takes his time, and lingers in exploratory pleasure. I encourage you to slow down and pay attention to your woman's responses. Learn to cultivate your complementary energy and enjoy your goddess's yin rhythms. Go at her pace, not yours.

If you're disinclined to do this for her sake, do it for yours. The more you dance to her rhythm, the more you'll be rewarded.

Men, here's another reason to cultivate your complementary yin energy. By doing so, you can learn to expand your arousal and orgasm. Did you know that you can learn to channel your sexual energy away from explosive ejaculatory orgasm and send it up your spine? It's worth it, believe me (assuming, of course, that you'd like to find out what a full-body multiple orgasm feels like!). When you slow down and channel your goal-directed arousal, you'll find there's a new and wonderful sexual journey to enjoy.

Journey to the Origin of the World

"*This is the nucleus—after the child is born
of woman, the man is born of woman;
This is the bath of birth—this is the merge of
small and large, and the outlet again,
Be not ashamed, women—your privilege encloses
the rest, and is the exit of the rest;
You are the gates of the body, and you
are the gates of the soul.*"

—WALT WHITMAN

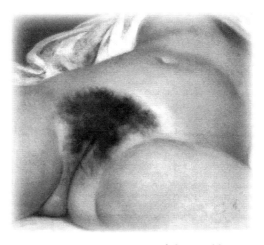

Gustave Courbet—*Origin of the World, 1866*

CHAPTER FIVE

Welcome to the Yoniverse

"To see you naked is to recall the Earth."
FEDERICO GARCIA LORCA

First Stop . . . The View from the Yard

OUR TOUR PROCEEDS FROM THE OUTSIDE to the inside for two reasons. First, it's always good to start with what you already know, so we begin

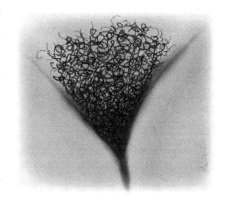

with the most familiar territory—the outside of the vulva. Second, this pathway, from outer to inner, recapitulates how feminine or yin sexual energy moves, and therefore is usually the pattern you'll want to use in the progression of your play.

We begin our journey with the outside of the crotch. For the many women who don't have female partners and who only see the casual nakedness of a locker room or sauna, all that's discernible in the flesh is the furry (or fur-free) triangle between the legs. Unless you get to enjoy intimate female parts in person, any close-ups you get will come from porn, a sex book or a textbook.

Unfortunately, the porn model of genital beauty is as limited as the fashion-model standard of how women's bodies should look. Still images are frequently air-brushed and photoshopped. In movies, the performers sometimes have their labia glued open for improved visibility. In addition, some of these women have had plastic surgery to look the way they do.

The sex book and textbook standard isn't much better, usually showing a diagram of a non-existent, generic, average white girl's version of the vulva.

GUIDED TOUR
Overview of Your Homeplay Assignment

I mentioned this earlier, and I'm repeating it here because it's so important. I advise you to do your homework (er, I mean homeplay!) in three stages:

1. NON-AROUSAL

- Begin in a state of non-arousal.

- Go on a tour and thoroughly check out all the parts described in the guided tour.

2. MEDIUM AROUSAL

- Play with yourself until you get to a medium level of arousal.

- Stop pleasuring yourself and take time to look at and feel the various parts again.

- Notice all of the changes—size, shape, color, sensitivity, energy, heat.

3. HIGH AROUSAL

- Play with yourself some more and get to high-level "Oh, oh, oh, I'm almost coming" arousal (or as high as you can).

- Stop again (yes, I know it's hard to stop, but it's worth it).

- Now, with the whole system fully turned on, check it all out again. You should be able to feel almost everything at this stage. Once again, notice all the changes—size, shape, color, sensitivity, energy and heat.

- Appreciate your transformed genitalia.

Trust me—you'll find that your body has done amazing things!

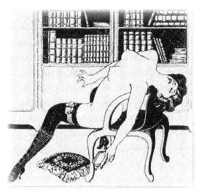

Setting the Stage (What You'll Need)

Before you get started, here's a list of goodies you'll need to make your sexploration the wonderfully positive experience it can be:

- Time, space and privacy

- Comfort and warmth

- Light (preferably free-standing, bendable neck lamp)

- Mirror (preferably magnifying)

- Your favorite sex toys and lubricant

- This book's GUIDED TOUR sidebars

- Courage (the antidote to fear)

- Curiosity (it won't kill your pussycat—it will awaken her!)

- Permission (you have to give it to yourself)

- Optional:

    Plastic speculum
    Drawing material
    Notebook and Journal
    Camera

THE GUIDED TOUR
Preparing For Your Journey

To get the full benefit of this tour, you'll need to follow along at home.

I strongly encourage you to make the time and create the space to really devote yourself to this journey of discovery. You can make this a special and even sacred exploration. Make sure you have the privacy you need. Do whatever is required to be uninterrupted. You'll also need to be comfortable and warm.

You can learn a lot just by feeling, but you'll get more out of your tour if you also look at the parts. For that, you'll need a light and a mirror. A large magnifying mirror will allow you to see all the delightful details. An adjustable goose-neck lamp is good to illuminate the vistas. In the ideal set-up, you'll place the mirror between your opened legs and shine the light on the mirror.

If you want to take the extra-credit side trip to see the beautiful inner caverns, you'll need a speculum and some nice lubricant.

If you don't want to go here on your own, the next time you're getting a gynecological exam, ask your care provider for a mirror and light and have them show you what they get to see. (Any good practitioner will be happy to help you learn about your body this way.)

This is your own personal sex tour (not the icky kind!) and includes the changes that happen when you get all turned on and juicy, so have your favorite sex toys (vibrator, erotica, lube, feathers, boy toys) close at hand. Many of the most wonderful parts of your genital system will only become evident when they're aroused, producing the delightful swelling called engorgement.

What this means is that you'll have to play with yourself to discover everything you've got. Once you find and feel all of the parts you really have, no one will ever be able to tell you differently. You'll have become your own anatomy expert and personal pussy authority.

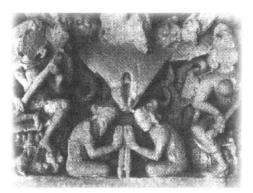

Sixty-Four Yogini Temple at Bheragat, India

Delicious Diversity and Vulvic Variety

Genitalia are as delightfully diverse as faces. Everyone has the same features—two eyes, a nose and a mouth—yet we all look distinct. All women have the same parts, but those parts can look extraordinarily dissimilar. The range of normal is much, much wider than most people think. Pussies are like flowers (which, after all, are the sexy bits of plants). The array is vast and the variations are what make them so beautiful, glorious and unique.

Before we embark on our inner tour, let's pause to appreciate a variety of normal, healthy and diverse vulvas.

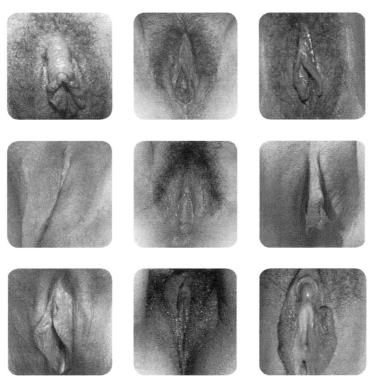

The Vulva Gallery—*The diversity of size, shape and color is only hinted at in these photos. The range of normal is enormous.*

The Voluptuous Vulva

Vulva is an inclusive term that includes all of the external parts of the yoni. While the female genitals are often incorrectly referred to as the vagina, that's only one portion of the equipment. We'll get to the vagina later, but for now let's stay and play with the *vulva*.

The Yard, Porch and Inner Sanctum

It is useful to think of the female genitalia as having three concentric zones. Imagine a lush garden surrounding an inviting portico that leads into a beautiful temple:

- YARD: the vulva, mons and outer lips are the "garden" or "yard" of the genitalia—the parts that are accessible from the outside.

- PORCH (A/K/A VESTIBULE): this includes the soft sensitive inner labia, the head of the clitoris and the delicate openings of the vagina, urethra and anus.

- INNER SANCTUM: The vagina and anal canal are your sacred, innermost areas.

THE GODDESS GUIDE
Claim Your Sacred Temple

To make your experience a spiritual journey, you can do your home-play as a ritual. Do whatever inspires a sense of the sacred for you.

Consider preceding the tour with a ritual candle-lit bath scented with essential oils. You may want to create a sacred space by lighting candles and incense. Surround your bed with flowers. Place special objects around you. Put on music that inspires you.

You can recite self-love mantras as you discover and venerate each wondrous part of your sacred anatomy. Utter affirmations of delight as you explore and connect with each amazing aspect. Some examples: "My yoni works wonderfully." "My pussy looks beautiful and smells delicious." "My clitoris is a sensitive jewel." (Or how about, "My anus is a holy hole?" Laughter is sacred, too!)

You can intersperse your tour with chants or sacred songs. Take time to practice ecstatic breathing. Draw a picture or take photos, then place them on an altar honoring your yoni.

If you feel so inclined, say words of protection or healing. You are, after all, the guardian of your gate. She needs to trust you to protect her. (If she doesn't, you may find yourself getting infections or having pain or other problems as she takes over the role of guardian.)

If you're a survivor of abuse, a commitment to being a fierce guardian of your gate is especially important.

If you have ever allowed anyone entry when it didn't feel right or good, consider making a vow to your yoni. What does she need to hear? Quite possibly this: "I will never allow anyone to enter you unless it feels great, unless all of me wants it, unless it's safe." Repeat as needed!

When you're done, you may want to journal or make art about your experience.

HOT TIPS FOR GUYS

To Get a Sex Goddess in Your Bed, Treat Her Like One

YOU ARE A LUCKY MAN to get to do your homeplay with this woman. Appreciate your partner's willingness to share this intimate journey.

Make a ritual of discovering your female friend's genitals. Honor her most delicate parts. Anoint her with coconut oil. Learn Tantric yoni massage and give her the gift of non-sexual pussy love.

Offer her worshipful adoration. Say mantras and affirmations of love, appreciation and positive regard such as, "I love all of you," "I delight in your beautiful yoni," "Your pussy is gorgeous," and "I love your scent." Women need oodles of positive pussy praise to get over our cultural messages of shame and disgust. Pile on the yoni worship!

Sit and gaze adoringly at her yoni. Bring it (and her) flowers. Place your hands over the entire area and send love energy into her as she breathes it in.

Ask before entering. Say "please." And remember: a heartfelt "thank you" is always appreciated!

The Outer Banks—The Mound of Venus

As we approach the outer banks, the first sight we see is the *mons*. Named for the goddess of love, your *Mound of Venus* forms a delta between your thighs, its hair-covered skin overlaying a pad of fatty tissue, providing a pubic-bone bumper. Prior to the current fashion of trimming and shaving, the furry outer triangle was all you could see when nude. Now that depilation has become popular, we may occasionally glimpse a bit more.

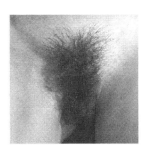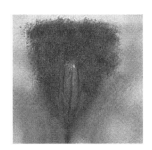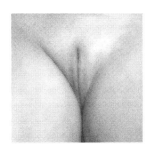

The Delta of Venus—From hair to bare.

The skin of the mons isn't especially sensitive, although it's connected to many other deliciously responsive bits. What it does have is an abundant supply of scent glands. Although our super-hygienic culture does its best to hide these odors, many primal animal sex signals are mediated by scent. It's one reason we still have abundant hair around our crotch and armpits. We produce scent for a reason: the smell is supposed to be sexy. Hair is there to capture our luscious aroma and thus reel in our suitors by the nose. The hair is also a clear marker of sexual maturity.

The Luscious Labia

With the next stop on our tour, just south of the mons, we come to the *labia majora*, meaning the "large lips." Calling them the *outer lips* or *external labia* is a more accurate name that fits every woman's body. They come in many varieties—from abundantly ample to provocatively plump to slender and svelte.

The outer lips form two fleshy parentheses that enclose and protect the delicate parts within. They're covered by regular external integument

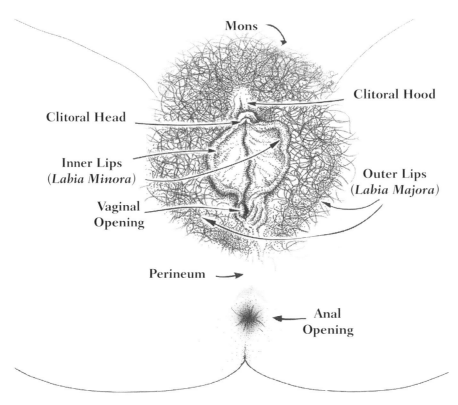

Mons

Clitoral Hood

Clitoral Head

Inner Lips
(*Labia Minora*)

Outer Lips
(*Labia Majora*)

Vaginal
Opening

Perineum

Anal
Opening

*A **Real Vulva**—Bottom View. This illustration shows the parts of a real vulva, which often doesn't reveal what's between the inner lips.*

(a fancy word for skin) and typically sport varying amounts of pubic hair. Beneath the skin, fatty tissue provides some padding.

They're not generally considered an especially sensitive area, but later on, when you learn what's under them, you may revise your view of their erotic potential.

Nestled inside the outer lips, you'll see the *labia minora*, meaning the "small lips." Since they vary so greatly in size, *inner labia* or *inner lips* is a more inclusive name.

For some women the inner lips are small, thin and dainty—you'll need to spread your outer lips to see the sights. For women with large flamboyant inner lips, they'll be quite visible without assistance as the elaborate folds and drapes of luscious inner lip tissue can protrude quite far from the outer ones. The two inner lips may be the same on both sides or quite different from each other. For most women, even with your legs spread open, the outer and inner labia together tend to enclose the rest of your tender parts.

The color ranges through the spectrum from delicate pink and salmon to tan and the darkest browns. The hue may be consistent or vary from area to area. The inner lips contain blood vessels that swell

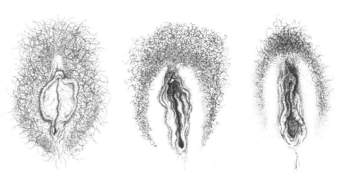

Labial Diversity—
Inner lips can vary
from small to large,
simple to elaborate,
symmetrical or un-
even—and all are
normal.

during arousal, so whatever color they begin with will darken as they infuse with blood. Again, the variations in color, size, shape, symmetry and sensitivity are normal. Size does not matter—it has nothing to do with your pleasure potential.

The Slippery Bits

The inner lips are covered with soft, moist delicate tissue called *mucus membrane* or *mucosa*. The slippery, silky mucosa covers all the structures that comprise the "porch," the vestibule area that's the middle ground of the female genitalia. The mucosa is seriously sensitive—it's easily irritated by contact with anything dry or rough as well as by the harsh chemicals of modern over-enthusiastic hygiene. In addition, vigorous erotic activities can rub this moist fragile membrane the wrong way. All that glistens on the porch is lubricious tender tissue and best touched by the wet and slippery.

HOT TIPS FOR GUYS
Slippery When Wet

Everything inside her outer lips is made of delicate mucus membrane, moist sensitive tissue that is designed always to be wet. Always touch this tissue wetly! Use lube, her own natural juice or saliva, but always moisten whatever you're using to touch her there. Her sensitive pussy porch is like the inner surface of your eyelid. Any contact with something dry, or worse yet, rough or (egad!) dirty will be irritating.

Play around with the outer surfaces of her vulva for a while. Not only will it heighten her arousal and drive her to wet wildness, but you can touch her in the yard with your dry fingers without worrying about accidentally rubbing her the wrong way. Remember, once you cross the threshold onto her porch, everything needs to feel slick and slide-y. Add more slippery stuff as needed!

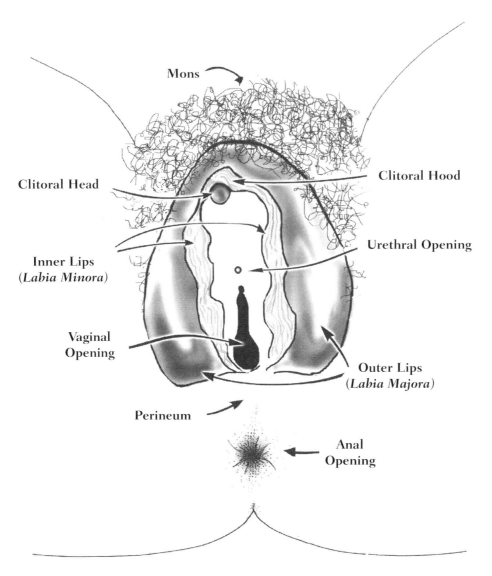

Mons

Clitoral Head

Clitoral Hood

Inner Lips
(***Labia Minora***)

Urethral Opening

Vaginal Opening

Outer Lips
(***Labia Majora***)

Perineum

Anal Opening

*A **Diagram of the External Vulva**—Bottom View. This diagrammatic view of the vulva reveals everything that can possibly be seen from the outside.*

Visiting The Vestibule

Once you're past the outer lips, you're in the *vestibule*. This is the porch of the pussy. As you spread the lips open, you'll see a variety of structures, including the opening to the vagina. We'll visit this doorway and the inner sanctum of the yoni later, but for now, let's hang out on the porch and see what else is there.

Above the vaginal orifice is the opening of the *urethra*, officially known as the *meatus* and more commonly referred to as the "pee hole." The urethra is actually the entire two to three-inch tube that exits from the bladder, transporting urine out.

In illustrations, the opening is often shown as a round hole located midway between the top of the vaginal opening and the head of the clitoris. In real women, it's rarely an obvious open hole—it's usually a small slit hidden between folds of tissue. It may actually be slightly in or just above the vaginal opening.

The opening of the urethra is quite sensitive and easily irritated, so direct contact absent arousal is best avoided. Later on, you'll learn when and why that changes.

HOT TIPS FOR GUYS
Supplicant at the Sacred Temple

When approaching a woman sexually, whether it's over dinner or in the bedroom, remember that her core yin energy needs to be aroused by starting at the edges and working your way in. You want her to bloom open like a flower. Think of it as a pilgrimage to a sacred temple where the journey is as important as the destination. Begin the trip by taking the time to connect with her emotionally, energetically and physically. Delight and awaken her whole body. Only after you feel her open and sense her energy accumulating in her sex center should you turn your attention there.

Think of your partner as having concentric zones, with the innermost one your ultimate target. I invite you to imagine them as a seven-step stairway to heaven:

1. The outermost zone is your larger connection—the context and surroundings, and both of your energy fields.

2. The non-erogenous areas of her body—shoulders, calves, arms and so on.

3. The non-genital erogenous zones—lips, mouth, ears, neck.

4. The genital vicinity—thighs, butt, hips, lower back.

5. The yard—the vulva, mons and outer lips of the pussy. These are the parts of her genitalia that are accessible from the outside. Think of her outer lips and the mons as a garden that surrounds a temple— hang out there for a while before moving to the porch. There's a lot to appreciate and enjoy in the yard!

6. The porch (a/k/a the vestibule). This consists of the soft wet middle areas, specifically her inner labia, clitoris and the delicate areas around the vaginal and anal openings.

7. Her inner sanctums—inside the vagina and anus. (continued on next page)

You will delight your goddess the most when you move gradually, sensitive to her cues about pace, from the outer to the inner circles. Remember: it's not how fast you get to the target, but how slowly and patiently you can coax her flower to blossom and burst.

It's usually a good idea to play in the outer zones for a while before going in to the next level. In fact, I encourage you to stay out of her innermost zones until she actively urges you to go there. The inner temples of her vagina and anus are the last place her arousal energy gets to and thus the last place you should be visiting. Let her hunger precede your entrance.

If you want the magic door to this inner realm to fully and actively open for you, don't be in a rush to get there, and definitely don't go barging in. If you're a master lover, you'll wait until she's inviting (or better yet, begging) you to come inside! Remember that we goddesses always appreciate it when you ask if we're ready to receive you. Your reception will be warmest when we're eagerly opening for you. When you do enter her body, do it consciously, with exquisite attention. Even then, don't just plunge all the way in. Take your time and explore the area just inside the doorway. Let her avidly suck you further in. Sometimes driving her crazy is a good thing!

Openings and Orifices

From the yard, when you spread the yoni lips, you can see two holes, with a third, so to speak, behind. An "orifice" is medical lingo for a hole or opening. The southernmost opening is the *anus*, the orifice known far and wide as the asshole. Above that is the *vaginal opening*. Often referred to as the vagina (which actually means the whole canal), this orifice is usually not a gaping hole, but a crevice or crack between the drapes of the lips. Between the clitoris and the vaginal opening is the *urethral aperture*.

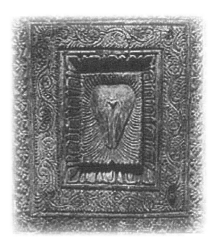

The Glittering Clitoris

At the top of the vulva we find the "jewel of the yoni," which in most books is referred to as the *clitoris*. More accurately, this is the *head*, also known as the *glans*, the acorn-

Vulva Carving, Ancient Temple in Thailand

shaped part that forms the tip of the three-piece clitoral network. Containing a remarkable 6,000–8,000 nerve endings, it richly merits the fame it's garnered as the epicenter of feminine delight. This is the highest concentration of nerve endings anywhere in the male or female body, making it uniquely and exquisitely sensitive. Most parts of the genitals are multi-purpose, but the clitoris is there for pleasure and pleasure only. Let's hear it for the bliss button!

> *"I stand in awe of my body."*
>
> HENRY DAVID THOREAU

Some clitoral heads are baby pea-sized, while others may be as big as an olive or as long as an inch or two. The diversity is wide and normal. Nub or stub, bitty button or proud protuberance, size matters not at all.

There's lots of variety in what gets women off, but it's safe to generalize that many if not most women need some form of targeted clitoral action to reach their orgasm. For some women, only direct stimulation will do, while others can climax with indirect attention. There are certainly women who can naturally orgasm from a variety of other stimuli (including but not limited to intercourse), although for most women these are acquired skills.* That said, it's still the case that clitoral play, even for advanced

---

* It's also true that every woman, including you, can learn to come from almost anything, over time, with lots of practice.

practitioners of the erotic arts, will usually be the easiest and most essential orgasmic trigger.

There's much more to come when we learn about the rest of the clitoris, but we'll get there later when we explore all of the sexy subterranean structures. First, though, let's see all of the sites in this locale before we go down.

The Handy Hood

The glans is nestled underneath a fold of skin called the *hood* that protects the clit's many thousands of nerve endings. This is similar to the foreskin of the male penis. The hood is formed by the joining of the top of the labia on either side. Because of this, when the lips are moved, there is indirect stimulation of the clit and the structures underneath the lips. That clever Creator! Not only do labia come in all colors, shapes and sizes, but there also are virtually endless variations in hood size, shape and color, as well as in how it attaches to the labia and the clitoral head.

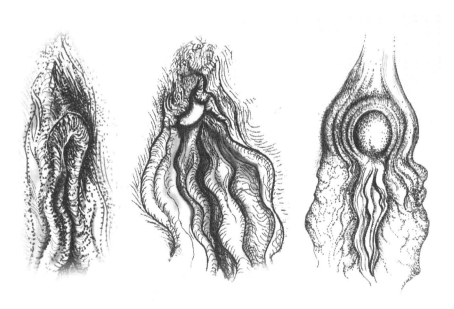

Clitoral Close-ups—*There are innate variations in how much the hood covers or reveals the clitoral head, from hidden to partially peeking to utterly out.*

In images, the clitoral head is almost always exposed, but in real women the arrangement varies enormously. Some clits are retiring, entirely covered by their hood when at rest. Some peek out a bit while others flaunt themselves audaciously. During arousal, the head usually retreats under the hood, but again, your mileage may vary. This has no

impact on your ability to have an orgasm: it matters not at all whether
you have an exhibitionist clit or a shy one when it comes to coming.

Hymen Today, Gone Tomorrow

At birth and throughout childhood, a thin membrane, called the *hymen*,
partially covers the vaginal opening, protecting it from infection. Sometimes the hymen is torn or stretched during childhood by accident or
activity. As girls become women, the hormones of puberty cause the
hymen to get thinner and it often disappears entirely, without any help
from pushy visitors. Other women have very stretchy hymens that remain
even after puberty and repeated vaginal penetration. What this means
is that, our longstanding cultural myth notwithstanding, the absence
or presence of the hymen is not a giveaway to newly-minted husbands
(or anyone else) about whether a woman has had prior intercourse or
penetration of any kind.

For most women, small hymeneal tags remain that fringe the inner
part of the vaginal opening.

A pervasive myth is that the hymen will painfully tear and bleed pro-
fusely during a woman's first experience of insertion. This is actually the
exception! If there *is* blood, it's usually just a few spots. Unfortunately, it
is the case that many women's first experience of intercourse is painful
and unpleasant, but you can't blame the hymen for that. Typically, the
discomfort arises from a lack of adequate arousal as well as not feeling
safe or as if they're acting with free choice during the experience.

Perineum—It Taint Nothing

The *perineum* is the area of smooth skin between the vaginal opening and the anus. The actual surface of the perineum has far fewer nerve endings than the rest of the genitalia as it is designed to take both the friction, rubbing and thrusting of intercourse and the remarkable stretching required for the emergence of a baby's head should that happen nine months later. It's actually a good thing that it's tough and flexible, but not acutely sensitive. Due to our medical culture's unfortunate training and belief system, many women who've had vaginal births have a scar along their perineum from an episiotomy, a surgical cut that is used during birth to help get the baby out

> *"Attending births is like growing roses. You have to marvel at the ones that just open up and bloom at the first kiss of the sun, but you wouldn't dream of pulling open the petals of the tightly closed buds and forcing them to blossom to your time line."*
>
> GLORIA LEMAY

a little bit faster. Since Mother Nature actually designed the vagina and perineum to be able to stretch open without surgical intervention, it's usually an unnecessary and occasionally harmful procedure.

For most women, the resulting scar tissue isn't a problem, but sometimes there's damage to the underlying erectile structure, muscles or nerves. When there is nerve damage, it can make the area numb or overly sensitive. In addition, scar tissue doesn't stretch, sometimes causing discomfort with penetration. This is yet another example of the miracle of modern medicine not being all that miraculous.

In some quarters, the perineum has the less-than-charming moniker of the "taint"—since it 't'aint the pussy and it 't'aint the asshole. It's also called the landing strip, for obvious reasons.

Just south of the yoniverse lies the oft-insulted and ignored anus. Lest you think we're skipping that delightful destination, let me reassure you—we'll return to the butt later.

An Acquired Taste

Appreciating the scent and taste of our partners' genitals is natural for some and an acquired taste for others. The bouquet of your partner's parts can be a huge turn-on. We are designed to desire, and scent is a natural and primary lust-enhancing device. As for being on the receiving end of lingual love, there's nothing hotter than an enthusiastic partner who loves your scent and flavor and lets you know it.

Each of us has our own unique, natural, sexy, spicy bouquet. Female genitalia are not supposed to smell like fake flowers or perfume, and despite the familiar cultural reference, they don't smell like fish either, not even high-grade sushi tuna. On the contrary, a bad (as distinguished from musky) odor is a sign of imbalance or infection and requires healing, not deodorizing. A healthy pussy doesn't smell or taste bad. Yes, our muffs are musky . . . and delicious!

CHAPTER SIX

An Erector Set of Her Own

*"Our own physical body possesses a wisdom
which we who inhabit the body lack."*

HENRY MILLER

Going Underground

WE'RE ABOUT TO DESCEND INTO THE PARTS that can't be seen with the naked eye, no matter how naked we may be. Imagine that we're going under the skin, fatty tissue and top layer of muscles to reveal an exquisite treasure awaiting discovery. Yes, this is where you'll find "buried pleasure!" The riches we'll bare include the systems and structures that make up the elegant female erectile network.

First, though, let's take a moment to study, understand and appreciate what is in essence a great cultural secret: women have an erector set of their own.

Men Get Erections, Women Get . . . Herections!

Erectile tissue is a unique type of tissue consisting mostly of a compacted mass of specialized capillaries. Capillaries are the tiniest blood vessels in

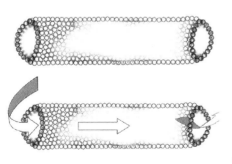

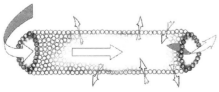

the body with a wall only one cell thick. You have regular capillaries all over your body, supplying each and every tiny cell. The thin wall allows for exchange to occur, enabling our bodies to absorb things like oxygen and nutrients and to eliminate wastes.

A Regular Capillary—Capillaries are our tiniest blood vessels. Top) This super close-up of a regular capillary shows the single-cell wall. Middle) Blood flows through. Bottom) The thin wall allows for exchange to take place.

Erectile tissue, however, boasts some very unusual and talented capillaries that are endowed with an extraordinary feature: they have a multitude of miniscule one-way valves. When you're not aroused, they stay open, allowing blood to flow just as in regular circulation. When you get turned on, the valves cooperatively close, allowing the tissue to fill up with blood. It's not unlike what happens when you stop up the drain at the bottom of your bathtub, but still have the faucet on. Blood continues to flow into the one-way passage, but it can't get out.

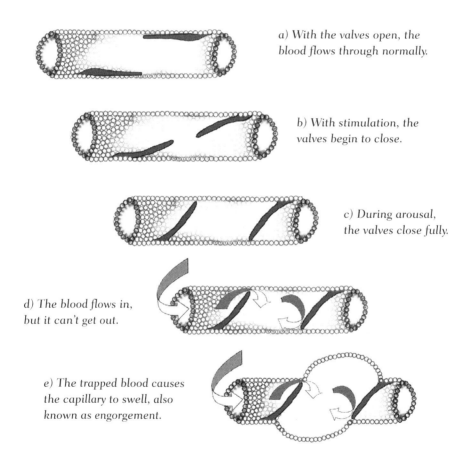

a) With the valves open, the blood flows through normally.

b) With stimulation, the valves begin to close.

c) During arousal, the valves close fully.

d) The blood flows in, but it can't get out.

e) The trapped blood causes the capillary to swell, also known as engorgement.

An Erectile Tissue Capillary—Erectile tissue is formed from specialized capillaries with structures that act as one-way valves.

There's something else that's special about erectile tissue, too. Some of it has balloon-like extra spaces where you can pack even more red-hot blood, increasing that extra-stiff feeling. When the erectile capillaries fill, the tissue becomes enlarged, firm and wonderfully sensitive, producing the delightful state called engorgement. Women have an entire network of structures composed of this wondrous, expandable erectile tissue.

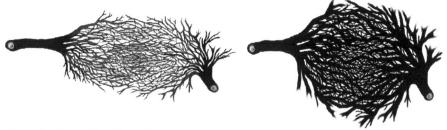

Erectile Tissue Capillary Network
Left: When not engorged, the erectile tissue capillary network is small. Right: When filled with trapped blood during engorgement, the erectile capillary network gets substantially larger (and firmer, darker and hotter, too.)

Similar But Not the Same

Erectile tissue in men and women is identical, although how it's laid out is quite dissimilar. *Vive la différence!* The penis essentially works as a single unit, with the action of all those clever valves coordinated. This enables men to maintain an erection and then to release all the valves in concert, providing force for their ejaculation. Following ejaculation comes the inevitable, inescapable refractory period, the time that must pass before a man can get erect again. Essentially, after all the valves release, they roll over and go to sleep. It's a pattern you may recognize.

Women don't need a propulsive ejaculation, so their tiny valves don't require coordinated effort. In addition, the female arousal network isn't one functional unit—it's got different compartments that can work together or independently. Women have no refractory period.

Once a woman has developed her orgasmic proficiency, learning to have prolonged and multiple orgasms can be a relatively easy next step. This is because there's no period of generalized collapse to get through. Because those spasms can be generated sequentially, they can keep on coming . . . and coming . . . and coming.

Men are different. While they usually have no problem accessing their orgasmic ability, it's more difficult for them to learn to separate orgasm from ejaculation, which is what they need to do if they want to have lots of orgasms without a refractory period.

The Exquisite Erectile Network

Now that you understand what erectile tissue is and how it works, let's get back to our regularly scheduled tour. Allow me to introduce you to the *erectile network*, the center of women's arousal system.

Women's erectile network is made up of the interconnected but separate structures of the clitoris, vestibular bulbs, and two sponges:

- The clitoris is composed of three parts—head, shaft and legs.

- The paired vestibular bulbs are shaped like fat parentheses around the vaginal opening, lying under the lips.

- One tubular sponge of erectile tissue surrounds the urethra that lies above the roof of the vagina.

- Another erectile sponge is in the floor between the vaginal and anal canals.

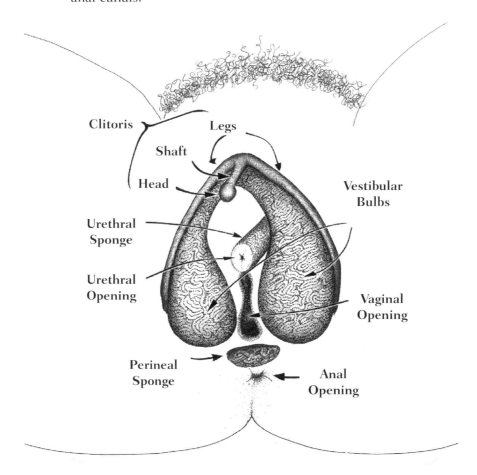

The Erectile Network and Associated Orifices—Bottom View. This is the same visual angle as the pictures of the vulvas seen in Chapter Five. These structures are under the skin, fatty tissue and top layer of muscles.

Each of these structures is linked to the others and designed to work in concert. This clever arrangement accords with Mother Nature's desire to ensure that reproduction is a pleasurable activity. Let's examine each of the structures in more detail to see how they work and to understand the ingenious connections of the sexual matrix.

Beyond the Button

We begin with a familiar part, the potent and super-sensitive clitoris, only now we'll explore all of it. Your entire clit, like the rest of your arousal network, is made up of that delicious magical substance, erectile tissue.

While many books show only the head, implying that it's the whole enchilada, the clitoris is actually composed of three parts, the *head* (also known as the *glans*, a name shared by the head of the penis), the *shaft* and the *legs*. We've already appreciated the clitoral head's wondrous sensitivity and delicate yet lusty nature. Now let's see where the rest of the clitoris is hiding.

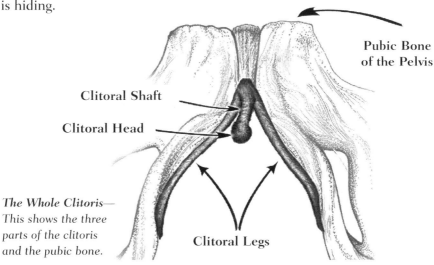

Pubic Bone of the Pelvis

Clitoral Shaft

Clitoral Head

Clitoral Legs

The Whole Clitoris—This shows the three parts of the clitoris and the pubic bone.

THE GUIDED TOUR
The Clitorati

*H*EAD AND HOOD: Beginning in an unaroused state, notice what your clitoral head looks like. Do you need to pull up on the hood to see it or does it show itself off? See how the lips attach and how your hood is formed. What happens when you tug at the lips—what else moves?

As you do your homeplay, notice how your clit changes at different levels of arousal. See and feel it as it becomes bigger, brighter, darker. Note how far up it moves as you get more turned on. As you play with your clit, notice how you may want more or less contact and different kinds of stimulation at various stages of arousal.

SHAFT: To find the shaft, place your fingers flat on top of the hood and feel the tubular structure beneath the skin. Roll it back and forth. You may want to pause and appreciate the sensations as you roll it from side

(continued on next page)

to side! This is a great move to get you started on the next phase of your home play by bringing you up to mid-level arousal.

Legs: You probably won't be able to discern much of the legs of the clit as they're commonly buried under too much tissue to be easily felt. At high-level arousal, you may be able to feel the top part of them. First find the base of the clitoral shaft and then move your fingers slightly apart and feel under the skin. The top part of the two ropey legs may be palpable when you're really hot and bothered.

HOT TIPS FOR GUYS
The Fabled Hot Button

You've all heard about how vitally important the clitoris is to female arousal. I applaud you for wanting to understand and attend to it. However, it's not a magic button that you can just press to get instant arousal or orgasm. The clit is sensitive, tiny and tricky. Pleasing it (and her) properly is a delicate matter.

For many women, the head of the clitoris is so sensitive that it can't be touched directly—or if so, only with great care. Remember, guys, this tissue is way more delicate than the tip of your tongue or fingertips.

The clit's sensitivity also changes as your partner's arousal level heats up. The hotter she is, the more likely it is that she'll want direct clitoral stimulation. Yet there can also come a time of extreme arousal when she becomes ultra-sensitive and less is more again. (I warned you, the clit can be very tricky!)

Once she's at mid-level arousal or higher, it's usually okay to move to direct genital play, but you may not want to start with the clit. If you go to her clitoris too soon or rub too hard, it will just be irritating and cause her to close up. If you're unsure, begin with tantalizing teasing and more generalized, inclusive stimulation. Continue with somewhat more indirect avenues to arousal.

Start with diffuse broad strokes, getting more focused as she gets hotter. Use your whole hand over the whole area. Play with the clit head and shaft through the hood or from the sides by grasping the outer lips and gently squeezing. Try frictionless rubbing of the shaft.

At high-level arousal, she may want (and, if you've really primed her pump, be begging for!) more direct clit attention. Wet, delicate and light will probably be her path to pleasure. Start slow and get faster but not harder, unless she asks for it.

This is an area that benefits from frequent check-ins. When you pay close attention to your pussycat's auditory and body-language signs of arousal, it will give you cues about to how to make her purr!

CLITORAL SHAFT

The head of the clitoris surmounts the tubular *shaft*, also known as the *body* or *corpus*. Covered entirely by the hood, the one-half to one inch-long shaft is about the width of a chopstick or pencil. It's surrounded by a loose tube of fibrous tissue, allowing some back-and-forth movement. You can easily feel it by placing your fingers on the skin of the hood and pressing down to feel it underneath. Try rolling it and rubbing happy little circles along its length . . . you'll like it!

"The clitoris is a phallus, atrophied in comparison with the male penis . . . this rudimentary organ is never destined to achieve . . . the degree of activity to which the penis can lay claim, for in this respect the male organ is far better endowed by nature."

MARIE BONAPARTE
Freudian Psychoanalyst

Together, the glans and the shaft are shaped like a tiny version of the cock. Anatomists have claimed that these two clitoral structures are analogous to the entirety of the penis. As you will see, they sadly underestimate the female equipment since these two pieces are only a small part of women's erotic equipment.

· ·

HOT TIPS FOR GUYS
Rolling the Shaft

Rolling the shaft is many women's favorite self-pleasure technique. The shaft is less likely than the head to get irritated and over-stimulated. Try back and forth movements or circular rubbing by pressing under the skin, stimulating it through the hood. You can also play with it indirectly from the yard, without worrying about the need to touch it wetly.

· ·

LUSCIOUS LEGS

The third part of the clitoris is much trickier to find and feel. At the base of the shaft, the clitoris bends and branches into two parts like a fat wishbone. The branches are called the *legs* or *crure* (crura is the singular). The four-inch legs follow along the inner edge of the pubic arch and anchor the clitoris—which fact, I suppose, gives an entirely new meaning to the term "leg man."

The legs are often difficult to find. You may feel the top part of them by spreading your fingers out and placing them on either side of the shaft and pressing down.

You've now been introduced to the complete clitoris—the head, the shaft and the legs. "Hello, clitoris, very pleased to meet you!" Remember: the entire clitoris, including the glans, the shaft, and the legs, is composed of erectile tissue, which means that the whole thing be-

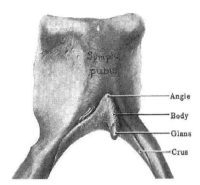

The Clitoris—This illustration is originally from the early 1900's. It shows the three parts of the clitoris and the attachment to the pubic arch of the pelvis.

comes enlarged, firm, and extremely sensitive with the right stimulation.

Hooray for the clitoris! There's a whole lot more to the female erectile circuits than that, though.

HOT TIPS FOR GUYS
Tender Touch Techniques

Most of the time, friction is not your friend (or hers). When you rub your fingers on her sensitive skin, it can be irritating. Lubricant can be useful if you're sliding over skin. Or, as an alternative, you might try using non-friction touch techniques. Place your fingers (or whatever) firmly on the skin and maintain contact while pushing downward, then rub what's under the skin. When her skin moves with your fingers, you can extensively stimulate the underlying structures without causing irritating friction. Just like with a penis, the top layer of skin can slide over the underlying parts and feel very, very good for a very long time.

The Enticing Entry—The Vestibular Bulbs

The next place to visit on our tour is one that you've probably never heard of, the *vestibular bulbs*. They're like a beautiful undiscovered beach—if everyone knew they were there, they'd be getting a lot more traffic!

The bulbs are two big wads of erectile tissue, nestled beneath the labial lips. These substantial teardrop-shaped structures lie on either side of the entrance or vestibule of the vagina, surrounding it like a pair of plump parentheses. They start on either side of the vaginal orifice and extend up along the sides. At the top, they connect directly to the shaft of the clitoris. (See *Erectile Network and Associated Orifices* on page 104.)

Hmmm….isn't that interesting! This connection means that when the bulbs are stimulated, so is the clitoris, and vice-versa. Not only that, but since the vestibular bulbs, like the clit, are made of erectile tissue, they'll get engorged when stimulated, whether directly or indirectly. When they puff up, the bulbs make the vaginal opening both expandable and a snug fit, enabling reproduction to work well with almost any male, regardless of his endowment. Convenient, eh? And this isn't Mother Nature's only evolutionary

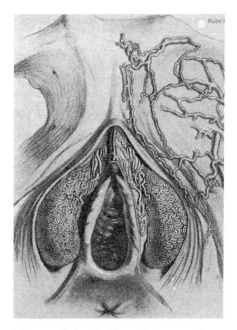

The Vestibular Bulbs and Associated Structures—This illustration from the late 1800's clearly and correctly shows the vestibular bulbs and associated structures. However, the gaping open vaginal orifice is not anatomically correct.

strategy vis-à-vis the bulbs. Since they're erectile, they make intercourse more pleasurable for women, and this makes them likelier to do the deed that makes more babies.

Not knowing about the existence or function of the bulbs is one reason some women don't enjoy penetration. It also helps explain why only about half of women experience orgasm during intercourse. If you're having vaginal penetration without big puffy bulbs, you're doing it before your body is really ready. Penetration simply won't feel great (or as great as it can feel) unless the bulbs are activated and sweetly swollen. When they're really big, it feels delicious to have something inside. I encourage you to pay attention to those bulbs and make sure they get the attention they deserve!

The bulbs are easily felt when engorged. Much like a penis, they increase substantially in size and grow quite firm as the erectile tissue fills with blood. With adequate stimulation, you'll have a distinct "hard-on" (or, rather, "hard-around") as the bulbs form a tumescent cuff around most of the vaginal opening when fully activated. When they're properly puffed, you should have a generous handful of plump pussy to play with—your very own herection!

THE GUIDED TOUR
Blossoming Bulbs

*L*ook at the area around the opening of your yoni, under the outer and inner lips when you're not turned on. Place your fingers firmly on the skin on either side of your vaginal opening and press down, feeling through the skin and fatty tissue to the muscles and bulbs beneath them.

Start to rub your bulbs and you'll feel them swell up under your fingers like the Pillsbury dough boy (or girl, in this case). Explore the different ways you can rub, squeeze and stimulate them, discovering what inspires them to enlarge.

Do whatever works to move you through your arousal journey, including intermittently playing with your clitoris. But keep returning to your bulbs to appreciate their transformation. As you move through the three stages of your homeplay (not aroused, moderately so and very hot), you'll discover just how big your hard-a-round can get!

When it's really puffy, you can easily feel the shape of each bulb, which is fat at the bottom and thin as it proceeds up towards the clitoris. Put one finger just inside your vagina and press toward the side to feel the rounded inner surface of the bulb. Add another finger on the outer side of the outer lip and squeeze to feel the plump rounded shape of the lower half of each bulb. This is a great time to take a look in the mirror and notice how the whole shape of your vulva is altered by the blooming bulbs. Enjoy!

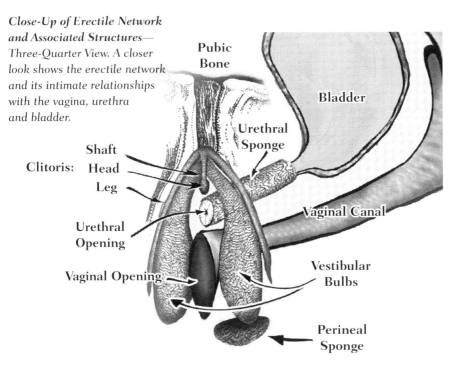

Close-Up of Erectile Network and Associated Structures—Three-Quarter View. A closer look shows the erectile network and its intimate relationships with the vagina, urethra and bladder.

Pubic Bone

Bladder

Shaft

Clitoris: Head

Leg

Urethral Sponge

Urethral Opening

Vaginal Canal

Vaginal Opening

Vestibular Bulbs

Perineal Sponge

HOT TIPS FOR GUYS

Puffing and Plumping the Bulbs

The outer lips are frequently ignored as a pleasure zone and mainly thought to be there to protect the delicate parts within. Guys, don't overlook them! You can play with those juicy vestibular bulbs from the yard, that is, through the outer surface of the outer lips.

Start genital stimulation with wide, diffuse, firm touch to the whole yard or external parts of the vulva. Use your whole hand or a nice round thigh to press and push against the outer lips which overlay the area of the bulbs. All this can be done with clothes on. But don't neglect these lovely moves when the clothes come off.

Since the bulbs are the outermost area of the erectile network, and since female arousal tends to flow from the outside towards the inside, for most women the bulbs are a great place to launch pussy play. Direct clitoral attention is likelier to be more welcome after the lips and bulbs have been attended to. Try using broad stimulation to the whole outer surface of the vulva, concentrating on what's beneath.

Squeeze the bulbs from the outside of the outer lips. Rhythmically rub them through the skin in a stroking or circling motion. Vibrate your hand or fingers on top of them.

When you feel the whole pussy swell up under your hand, just like that lovely feeling of a cock getting hard as you hold it, that means it's time to start attending to other areas of her yoni. I especially encourage you to make sure this area is firm and swollen before attempting to enter her.

Going On and Going In

Our next stop on our tour takes us to the parts of the erectile network that lie in the mysterious realms of the inner sanctum, the sacred magic yoni-verse. For homeplay reasons, we'll be going in to explore at the three stages of non-arousal, medium arousal, and full force turn-on. Please use plenty of lube for the first two stages! For educational purposes, I encourage you to make an exception to the "Don't put anything in your pussy unless it feels fabulous" guideline. When you're having sex play with yourself and others, please do follow this precept! Your pussy will thank you.

The Groove Tube, a/k/a the Urethral Sponge

For our first stop inside the inner sanctum, we enter the pussy portal, and reach up to the roof of the vagina. This area has been dubbed the *g-spot* after the Dr. Grafenberg, who supposedly discovered it.* Unfortunately his description of the area as a "dime-sized spot" is incorrect.

Hence this area is also called the *anterior* or *urethral sponge*. It's also known as the *female prostate*, since embryologically it's formed from the same tissue that becomes the prostate gland in men. In modern tantra, this area is called the sacred spot or, as a way to incorporate and reclaim the word g-spot, the "goddess spot."

This doesn't really resolve the nomenclature problem because the sponge isn't really a spot. Whatever you call it—the groove tube, squirt tube, goddess crest, roof ridge, or simply your sponge—it's a tube of erectile tissue that surrounds the urethral canal. This sensitive zone is located above the vaginal roof, along the mid-line, behind and under the arch of the pubic bone. To repeat: it isn't a spot, it's a cylinder of spongy erectile tissue, and you can feel its underside through the front part of the top wall of the vagina.: (See *Erectile Network and Associated Orifices* on page 104.)

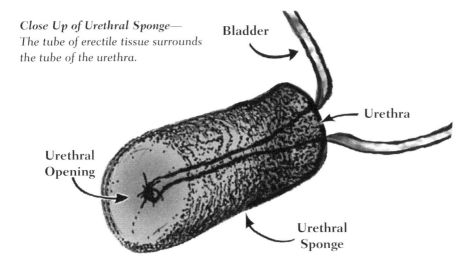

Close Up of Urethral Sponge—
The tube of erectile tissue surrounds
the tube of the urethra.

Bladder

Urethra

Urethral
Opening

Urethral
Sponge

Unlikely as it may seem, there continues to be some clinical and academic debate about whether this area exists, or if all women come equipped with one. Don't let that concern you, though. If you're female or have access to your lover's female parts, you should have no problem answering the question of the sponge's existence for yourself—and your answer will be in the affirmative.

---

* Historically, many female body parts have been named after the men who (supposedly) discovered them. That tradition is now seen as patriarchal, a form of colonizing women's bodies. This view makes sense to me. Why should the G-spot be named for a person who didn't have one?

The important thing to remember when seeking to confirm its existence is that it's composed of erectile tissue. When a woman is not aroused, there's not much there to feel. But when you are aroused, the spongy tube will change consistency and swell, like any good erectile tissue should. At that point, it's easy to feel the ridged tubular contour of the structure as well as the way it grows and becomes firm when turned on. When the sponge is properly attended to and well puffed, it will provide a lovely source of gratifying sensation, especially when there's something moving about inside the vagina. Or better yet, when something is directly and firmly stimulating the sacred cylinder itself.

THE GUIDED TOUR
The Succulent Sponge

Begin by putting one or two of your fingers inside and exploring your yoni. Your vaginal canal is lined with moist mucus membrane. To find your urethral sponge, turn the pads of your fingers up, curl them and reach up, exploring the roof of your vagina. The mucosa there is somewhat rougher then the smooth slick surfaces of your walls and floor.

Remember as you go on your guided tour that this is erectile tissue that you're feeling, so during stage one of your exploration, that is, in a completely unaroused state, it won't feel like anything in particular. Since the urethral sponge surrounds the urethra, when you push against the non-puffed tissue, you'll really be rubbing almost directly on your pee tube. It will probably make you feel like you need to pee. For most women, this is not an erotic sensation.

When you're moderately aroused, feel it again. Notice the differences in size and sensation. It probably won't feel irritating, but it may not feel great, either.

At this point, you may want to experiment with sponge play and see if you can feel it continue to swell under your fingers. Or, you may choose to return to pleasuring your clitoris and bulbs to bring you to high arousal.

Since this tissue is so deep inside, it'll respond best during the third stage of your exploration. Sponge play during high-level arousal is most likely to make you go, "Oh, yeah, that's what they're talking about!"

When your groove tube is really big and puffed, you'll be able to feel the whole two to three inch length of it. You'll also notice its ridged or ribbed texture. If you separate your fingers a bit, you can run them along the gutters or sides of the tube. If you can reach in far enough, you'll feel

(continued on next page)

where it ends. When you play with it for a while, you may notice that it starts to feel like a wet sponge, as if it's full of tiny fluid-filled grapes.

If you're using a mirror, you can see some interesting sights. If you hold your vagina open and look inside with a light, you'll see the roof bulging boldly down into your vaginal canal. You can also note the raised circular ring that's the end of the tube surrounding the opening of your urethra.

Since female arousal proceeds from outside to in, it makes sense that for most women, it doesn't feel good to have anything inside the vagina until the vestibular bulbs and the clitoris are turned on. Prior to a moderate level of arousal, stimulating the urethral sponge can be irritating. In fact, without engorgement, stimulation of that area will essentially be rubbing on the urethra itself and probably make a woman feel an urge to urinate. When a woman has reached a state of moderate or, preferably, high arousal and the tube has proceeded to puff, then sponge play becomes pure pleasure.

> *"I'll try anything once, twice if I like it, three times to make sure."*
>
> MAE WEST

HOT TIPS FOR GUYS

Stroking the Sponge

For most women, it doesn't feel good to have anything inside the vagina until all the external erectile tissue is well puffed-up first. The labia, the erectile tissue of the bulbs, and the clitoris need to be aroused before you enter her in any way. Wait until she's really hot and her pussy's plump and inviting you in.

The urethral sponge responds best to firm rhythmical rubbing and thrusting motions. Fingers are the best tool for the job of directly stimulating this area, at least to begin with. Try one or two, as she prefers. Try a come-here gesture, crooking your finger to stroke along the length of the tube. Play with a windshield wiper motion, rubbing firmly back and forth. Rhythmically press and release. With two fingers inside and your thumb outside, grip the whole area and vibrate your hand, starting small and getting more intense. Run your fingers along the gutters on either side of the tube. Reach back to the tail or end of the tube and pull it towards you. Use strong pressure and be consistent with your motions. You should feel the tissue get increasingly spongy as it swells and fills. Yum!

Infection Protection

The urethral sponge has several functions besides providing pleasure. It's there to protect the vulnerable urinary tract from invasion and infection. It does this in three ways. First, when properly puffed, it cushions the sensitive urethra from the mechanical battering and irritation of intercourse. Inflamed tissue is more vulnerable to infection. Second, when the sponge is engorged, it narrows the urethral opening, thereby decreasing the potential for invasion by microbes.

> *"There is more wisdom in your body than in your deepest philosophy."*
>
> **FRIEDRICH NIETZSCHE**

Last but not least, the urethral sponge houses the paraurethral glands, the source of female ejaculate. Although there is no scientific data about this, I believe the fluid is antimicrobial—there to prevent infections of the urinary system.

From an evolutionary perspective, this protection is vitally important. An untreated urinary tract infection (UTI) can easily ascend, leading to a more serious infection of the kidneys. That infection can rapidly proceed to a potentially fatal full-body infection called sepsis.

As many women who've suffered from a UTI know, these infections are often related to sex. After all, the urethra is quite vulnerable what with the proximity of the anus, our own germs on our own hands or toys, and of course, the potential invaders brought by otherwise friendly sexual visitors. The urethra sits smack-dab in the middle of a Grand Central Station for microbes. And then we make matters worse with our rubbing and grinding and pumping! It's no wonder urinary infections are so common in women.

All our orifices have immune structures in their vicinity to protect us from microbial threats. For instance, the mouth and nose have the tonsils, adenoids and lymph nodes nearby. Since Mother Nature planned on our having genital company, and with the prox-

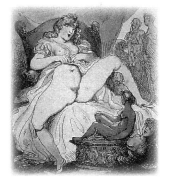

Thomas Rowlandson, c. 1800

imity of our waste-disposal system just to the south, it makes sense for her to have given us protective equipment near the vulnerable urethra. This appears to be the role of the paraurethral glands.

We'll return to this topic later when we get to the joy of squirting, but for now let's visit the rest of the fabulous erectile network.

The Fabulous Floor—The Perineal Sponge

We still have one more area to explore. (I'll bet you had no idea that such a treasure trove of puffy pleasure awaited you!) This next pad of erectile tissue is located under the floor of the vagina, beneath the perineum, in the wall between the vaginal and anal canals. This delightful territory, which has escaped the attention of pretty much everyone, sex experts and doctors alike, is called the *posterior* or *perineal sponge*, or *perineal body*. I also call it the *floor, bottom* or *rear sponge*. The perineal erectile tissue is usually one-half to one-and-a-half inches inside the vaginal opening and about one-half inch deep, towards the rectal wall. This depth tends to protect it from trauma during childbirth.

Again, like the other erectile tissue that forms the snug and sensitive cuff around the vaginal opening, evolution designed this tissue to best appreciate firm, rhythmical stimulation. (See *Erectile Network and Associated Orifices* on page 104.)

THE GUIDED TOUR
The Sponge in the Floor

To find your perineal sponge, put your thumb inside your vagina and push down towards your butt. First, go in about one-half inch and feel, then go another half-inch in, and then try one more little step inside. Somewhere in that range, you'll find your rear sponge.

Another way to feel your perineal sponge is to put your thumb in your pussy and a finger in your ass. As you bring the fingers together and proceed to move inward you'll find a fat area—yup, that's the spot! If you go in deeper, you'll have passed the mark and find that the rest of the wall between the two canals is quite thin and flexible.

When feeling your urethral sponge without arousal, you probably won't feel much. At mid-level arousal, it will be slightly firmer and more sensitive. At high-level turn-on, it will be quite distinct as a firm spongy yummy place to play with.

This brings us to the end of our exploration of the discrete set of structures that form the female erectile network. Our next stop will take us more deeply into the inner sanctums, including more of the vagina and that much-maligned pleasure palace, the anal canal. We'll also explore the rest of the multi-purpose female erotic equipment. On we go!

CHAPTER SEVEN

The Inner Sanctums

"If anything is sacred, the human body is sacred."
WALT WHITMAN

The Vital, Vigorous, Voluptuous Vagina

THE VAGINA IS A PASSAGEWAY formed by a pliable tube surrounded by layers of muscle. *Vagina* is Latin for sheath, as in a repository for a sword. Besides not finding it to be a particularly sexy word, it's an unpleasant image, yet another reason why I prefer "pussy" or" yoni."

The functions routinely listed for it are to provide a pathway for menstrual blood, a passage for semen, and an exit route for babies. It has another role, too, and it's an important one: it's there to produce fabulous sensations when filled and properly played with.

While it is often portrayed as being an open tunnel, this is one thing it is not. The vagina is a softly collapsed tube. The walls fold in and touch like a closed accordion. It's a truly remarkable structure due to its ability to contract and expand. Despite its appearance of being a rather small orifice, it can get big enough to birth an entire baby, and it can also contract enough to make a snug sleeve for any size cock. It's a remarkable multi-purpose instrument.

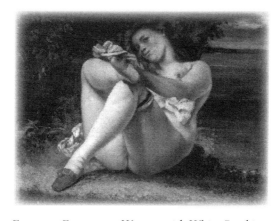

GUSTAVE COURBET—*Woman with White Stockings*

THE GODDESS GUIDE
Guardian of Your Gate

Women, I've mentioned this before, but it's so important it bears repeating. Never let anything enter your pussy before you're ready. Don't accept penetration of any sort unless it's feeling fabulous. It's your job to take care of yourself by being very attuned to your own readiness and response. Just because he's hard and ready doesn't mean it's time to let him in. Always pay attention to your own arousal and readiness and base what you do on that, not on your assessment of what he wants.

If you're already engaged in a particular act, especially intercourse, and it starts to feel less then wonderful, that's the time to end it. There are plenty of other sexy ways to play. If you're not getting off, if your arousal level is dropping, or if it's starting to irritate you or make you sore, call a halt to the proceedings immediately, if only temporarily. Your pussy (and your whole being!) will appreciate it.

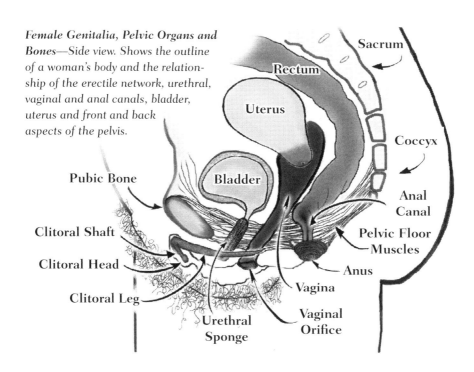

Female Genitalia, Pelvic Organs and Bones—Side view. Shows the outline of a woman's body and the relationship of the erectile network, urethral, vaginal and anal canals, bladder, uterus and front and back aspects of the pelvis.

Sacrum

Rectum

Uterus

Coccyx

Pubic Bone

Bladder

Anal Canal

Clitoral Shaft

Pelvic Floor Muscles

Clitoral Head

Anus

Clitoral Leg

Vagina

Urethral Sponge

Vaginal Orifice

The pussy's walls are lined with mucus membrane that produces slippery lubrication. There is always some vaginal lube present, but more is produced during sexual excitation. Vaginas of women who are either post-menopausal, post-partum or breastfeeding will be drier and more fragile. There is wide normal variation in lubrication depending on a woman's natural tendencies, where she is in her monthly cycle, and if she's taking artificial hormones or other medications. No matter who you are, or where you are in the cyclic life dance, having plenty of extra lube handy is always advisable.

HOT TIPS FOR GUYS
Prevent Premature Penetration

Increased vaginal lubrication is an early sign of arousal. Men often interpret this to mean she's ready to receive you in her pussy. Not necessarily! Just because she's wet doesn't mean she's ready for the insertion of anything. It may mean she's just getting started.

A woman's yoni is her innermost sanctum. Her yin arousal energy needs to accumulate there before she'll be ready to open fully and receive. Measure her arousal by the swelling of her erectile network and her body signs such as breathing, sound and movement.

In addition, there may be times when you need to take care of your partner because she's not taking care of herself. Many women are so out of touch with their own arousal level and so concerned with pleasing you that they will allow you to be inside them before they're ready. I encourage you to check in before entering. In fact, it's always a good idea to check in and ask if she's ready for whatever it is you want to do! She'll appreciate it and it's also a wonderful way to learn how to pleasure her.

If she's not ready for penetration or realizes that it's not feeling great after you're in, don't take it personally. If you are asked to go, do so immediately and graciously. Redouble your focus on her arousal and raise the heat until she's ready. It'll be a lot more fun for both of you.

When you honor your woman's yoni, it will release the goddess in her. Never enter her in any way until there's no question whatsoever about her wanting it!

The Self-Cleaning Vagina
The vagina is a delicate self-sustaining ecosystem. Treat your pussy well! Avoid all chemicals and products that can disturb her sensitive natural balance.

A Short Course in Vaginal Ecology

A healthy vagina is full of a special type of friendly normal bacteria, called *lactobacillus acidophilus*. These good bacteria protect the vagina and keep it healthy. One of their jobs is to control the population of unfriendly microbes such as yeast and "bad" bacteria. The pH (or acid-alkaline balance) in the vagina needs to be mildly acidic and normally varies slightly during the monthly fertility cycle.

If your healthy bacteria die off, unfriendly bacteria or yeast are free to take over. Taking antibiotics can cause your normal flora to die off. Exposure to chemicals and cleaning products can also shift the balance and cause a die-off of supportive bacteria. Sometimes it just seems to happen for no reason, with the hidden underlying cause being factors such as stress, poor diet or misguided "hygiene" practices.

Signs of infection include increased discharge above what's normal for you at that point in your cycle; any change in color or consistency; itching, pain or discomfort; or bad smells. Be on the lookout for these things! And don't abuse your pussy by buying into our cultural (and consumerist) obsession with hyper-cleanliness. Yes, it's good to be clean, and there can also be too much of a good thing.

Vaginal infections such as bacterial vaginosis (BV) and yeast (also known as candida or monilia) are often caused by over-enthusiastic and excessive hygiene. This includes the use of douches, vaginal deodorants, sprays, wipes, washes, powders, anti-bacterial soaps, deodorant soaps, body washes, bubble baths and so-called feminine hygiene products.

Spermicide can also cause problems for women. Nonoxynol-9 is the chemical name for this highly irritating substance. It's found on spermicidal condoms as well as in contraceptive jellies, foams and suppositories. Avoid it in any form.

Your healthy vagina tastes and smells savory and doesn't need irritating chemicals to be delicious. There is no need to clean inside the vagina at all, ever! You have a self-cleaning vagina.

It is normal to have vaginal discharge, indeed it is an essential component of the vagina's ability to keep itself clean. Normal discharge does not itch, burn, or feel irritating. It has a faint, pleasant, slightly musky odor. The discharge varies in color, consistency and amount depending on where a woman is in her fertility cycle, and whether she is on hormonal birth control or is post-menopausal. The color varies from white to clear. The amount ranges from scant to moderate. Some women are normally drier, while some tend to be wetter. It is important to know what amount is normal for you.

A Womb of Her Own

The *uterus* or *womb* is an amazingly strong multilayered organ shaped like a pear. It has multiple muscle layers and a remarkable lining capable of adapting to the cyclic changes of the fertility cycle. The *cervix* is the bottom part of the uterus—think of it as the smaller end of the pear. It nestles in the back of the vaginal canal. The opening to the uterus, called the *os*, is in the center of the cervix. Inside the cervix are microscopic glandular crypts that secrete a special slick mucus during the fertile time of a woman's cycle. These "sperm hotels" support the reproductive

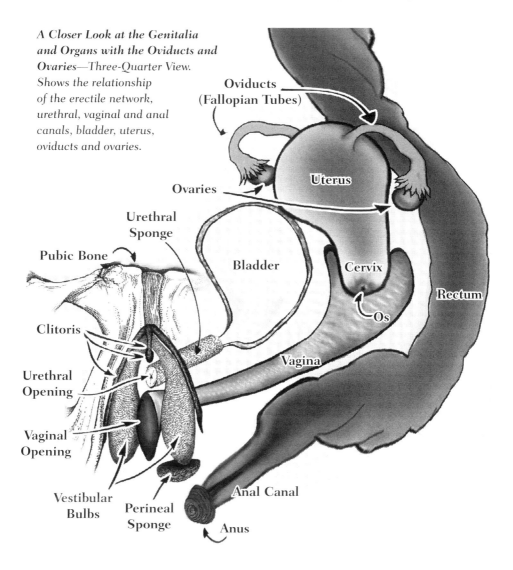

A Closer Look at the Genitalia and Organs with the Oviducts and Ovaries—Three-Quarter View. Shows the relationship of the erectile network, urethral, vaginal and anal canals, bladder, uterus, oviducts and ovaries.

Oviducts (Fallopian Tubes)

Uterus

Ovaries

Urethral Sponge

Pubic Bone

Bladder

Cervix

Rectum

Os

Clitoris

Urethral Opening

Vagina

Vaginal Opening

Vestibular Bulbs

Perineal Sponge

Anal Canal

Anus

process by keeping the sperm alive for up to five days as they await a forthcoming egg. The fertile mucus produced by these glands also acts like a slip-and-slide to help sperm on their journey into the uterus.

At either side of the top of the uterus are the two *fallopian tubes*, also known as the *oviducts* or *egg tubes*. At the end of each rests an *ovary*, the small pair of olive or almond-sized organs that contain all a woman's eggs. The ovaries nestle next to the uterus, not hanging out in space as depicted in many pictures.

REALLY ROUND LIGAMENTS?

Also on the top of the uterus is the pair of structures called the *round ligaments*, which aren't really ligaments at all.* They are actually a pair of long ropy muscles surrounded by a fibrous (or ligamentous) sheath. The round ligaments begin on either side of the top of the uterus and pass over the top of the pubic bone, with the far ends attaching to the muscle that encircles the opening of the vagina.

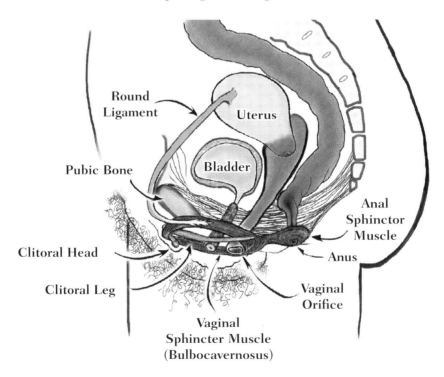

Female Genitalia and Organs with Round Ligaments—Side View. *Shows how the round ligament rises from the top of the uterus, crosses the pubic bone and inserts in the vaginal sphincter muscle known as the bulbocavernosus (the name reflects that it covers cavernous erectile tissue bulbs!).*

---

* Ligaments are structural, inelastic connective tissues that attach an organ, cartilage or bone to another bone.

GETTING IT UP

Based on the above, you'd almost think sexual arousal and reproduction have something to do with each other. And in fact they do. These so-called ligaments are responsible for the part the uterus plays in the female sexual response. That's right—the uterus is a player in the game of arousal and orgasm.

The uterus is not a fixed organ—it moves. It rises and falls, following a predictable pattern, during a woman's fertility cycle. When a woman is most fertile, the uterus rests highest up. When she's about to bleed or during her bleeding time, it sits lowest down. But the fertility cycle isn't the only cause of uterine movement. It also moves during arousal.

As a woman gets turned on, muscle tension increases, which causes the round ligaments to shorten. This action lifts the womb up and forward while pleasurably tugging on the muscular opening of the vagina. As the women's turn-on escalates, the womb is raised further and further up, like a taut bowstring being pulled way back. This also opens up a space at the back of the vagina, forming a nice cozy sperm-bowl and proving once again how clever Mother Nature is. It also pulls the cervix safely out of the way of any potential battering.

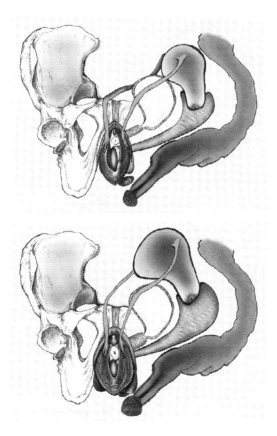

The Transformations of Arousal—Three-Quarter View. Notice the changes as the unaroused system on the top transforms into the aroused one on the bottom. The round ligaments shorten, pulling the uterus forward and up, resulting in expansion of the back of the vagina. The erectile network swells considerably. As it engorges, it forms a cuff that compresses the vagina, especially around the opening.

Now, here's the really good part: during orgasm, the uterus pulses up and down in a deep, slow, throbbing background rhythm that provides a bass counterpoint to the faster quivering of the pelvic floor muscles as they spasm. This pulsing adds emotional and erotic richness to the orgasm, and it also helps the uterus to suck up any sperm that happen to be hanging around in the nice open bowl at the back of the vaginal vault.

THE GUIDED TOUR

Follow the Bouncing Uterus (Extra Credit Homework)

You can notice how your uterus moves. If you're a woman in your fertile years and not on hormonal contraception, try sticking your finger in your vagina every morning for a cycle or two. You'll find that your cervix (the part of your uterus that pokes into the back of your vagina) is in a slightly different place every day. During your bleeding time, it will be low. After your bleeding is over, it will retreat until at ovulation it is farthest away from the entrance. After you ovulate, it will begin to descend again.

All women with a uterus can play with the changes in its position during the arousal journey. Reach in and feel it before you begin. Check again when you're moderately turned on. Feel once more as you get close to coming. You'll notice that it seems to be retreating. At that point, especially if you're in the fertile part of your cycle, you may not be able to reach your cervix at all. If you can keep your fingers deep inside during orgasm, you'll feel your cervix bobbing up and down and kissing your fingertips as you come.

Women who've had a hysterectomy (surgical removal of the uterus) often say their orgasm feels different. Although doctors often dismiss this complaint, saying that the problem is "all in their head," it's not. No uterus means no throbbing base counterpoint. It's a qualitatively different—and diminished—orgasm.

As most (but unfortunately not all) of us know, women can get pregnant without having an orgasm. This doesn't mean orgasms are irrelevant to fertility, though. If a woman wants to maximize her chances of making a baby, it helps if she has lots of rip-roaring orgasms to aid those eager swimmers on their way.

THE GUIDED TOUR

Boldly Go Where No Man Has Gone Before (Except Your Gynecologist)

*I*f you want to find out what your gynecologist or practitioner has been looking at every time you get a pelvic exam with a speculum, I encourage you to do so. I promise you, it's a worthwhile trip. In fact, it may be a great antidote to previous disempowering pelvic exams.

Make sure you have your light and magnifying mirror handy and that your speculum is warm. Practice opening and closing the speculum until you feel confident you know how it works. Also practice opening and closing your pelvic floor muscles.

When you feel confident that you can work all the equipment, lube up and insert the speculum with the handle up. (This is the opposite of how a practitioner would do it.) Breathe deeply and let your pelvic floor muscles relax and open. Let your mouth and face relax and open, too. Open the speculum, adjust your mirror, and position your light to shine on the mirror.

Now you can see how cool you really are inside. Notice the color of your inner walls. See the round pink donut of your cervix and the dimple of your os. If you rotate the speculum, you can see the rough, textured vaginal roof bulging downwards. Your urethral sponge is beneath it.

For extra credit, see if you can move your cervix by bearing down with an exhale.

We've All Got to Go Sometime

Any discussion of the inner sanctum would be incomplete without mentioning the *bladder*, which sits behind the pubic bone in front of the uterus. It's essentially a urine collection bag. From there, the pee is transported out of the body. This is the role of the urethra, which we met earlier in connection with the urethral sponge. The urethra provides the passageway for urine to exit the bladder. (See Illustrations: *Female Genitalia, Pelvic Organs and Bones* on page 118 and *A Closer Look at the Genitalia and Organs with the Oviducts and Ovaries* on page 123.)

The Nerve! (Well, Actually, the Nerves!)

The entire genital area is richly supplied with nerves, which transmit sensations and trigger movement. Erectile tissue is particularly well connected! Nerves are structured like a tree—a large trunk splits into two paired branches, which then divide into smaller and smaller units down to the tiniest twigs, called *nerve endings*. There are also *nerve bundles* that weave together multiple nerves.

Most textbooks only associate one set of nerves with sexual arousal. This isn't accurate—there are at least three pairs of sexual nerves. The one usually mentioned are the *pudendal nerves*, whose branches innervate the skin in the genital area, the three parts of the clitoris, the outer aspect of the urethral sponge, and most of the superficial pelvic floor muscles.

Etymologically, pudenda comes from the Latin *pudendum*, meaning "to be ashamed of." The word pudenda has also been used to refer to the entirety of the female genitalia. A less negative name would seem to be in order. Since it connects to the more superficial genital structures, I call it the *External Genital Nerve*.

A second set of nerves serving the genitalia are the *pelvic nerves*, which innervate the deep sexual structures with branches to the uterus, bladder, anus and the inner layers of the pelvic floor muscles. It also connects to the vestibular bulbs, the perineal sponge and the deeper part of the urethral sponge. (Note that the urethral sponge is delightfully connected to both nerve pathways!)

The pelvic nerves enter the vaginal area at the back of the vaginal vault. There the nerve bundles interweave into a *plexus* and then split into myriad smaller branches. In a non-aroused state, the cervix is usually in front of these areas. During arousal, the uterus moves up out of the

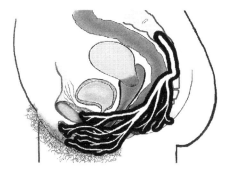

The External Genital Nerve—Side View. Shows the path of the pudendal or external genital nerve and the structures it innervates. These tend to be the more outer parts of the sexual equipment.

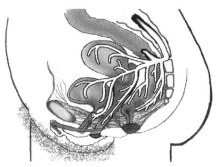

The Pelvic Nerve—Side View. Shows the path of the pelvic nerve and the structures it innervates. These tend to be the deeper organs.

way and exposes these spots, which can then be on the receiving end of powerful thrusting activity. At a time of high-level arousal, when the cervix is out of the way and the nerve plexi are available, 'pound, pound, pound' can be a very good thing.

If the woman isn't turned on enough to pull her uterus up, then deep thrusting will just knock into the cervix (ouch!), and it won't be pleasurable for her. This is another reason some women don't enjoy deep penetration or have orgasms from intercourse. Their cervix—and inadequate arousal—get in the way. These are the same spots that a baby's head hits as it descends into the birth canal, causing laboring women to spontaneously and powerfully push their infants out. Thus we have another example of evolution's design efficiency—the same powerful thrusting energy that got the baby started now helps get it out.

HOT TIPS FOR GUYS

A Pointer About Pounding

Guys, it's important to remember that not all nerves are created alike. The deep nerves are very different from the nerve endings that are part of the more sensitive erectile tissue, especially in the head of the clitoris and the mucosa around the lips and entrance of the vagina. It's great to pound when you're deep inside and your partner's at high arousal with her cervix pulled out of the way. With her more delicate nerve endings, it's better to stay delicate and subtle. They respond best to lighter tactile sensations such as caressing, light rhythmic motions and slippery rubbing.

Lastly, there are the *vagus nerves*, the wandering cranial nerves that originate in your brain and meander through most of your body, connecting to almost every major organ group. Its branches innervate the heart, the respiratory and gastrointestinal systems as well as the sexual and reproductive organs. The vagus nerves don't just connect multiple body systems. They also connect us to each other as they are part of our empathy system.

If you predominantly stimulate just one nerve pathway, you're likely to experience arousal and orgasm focused in its end-organ system. Thus stimulation of the structures innervated by the external genital nerve tends to lead to more clitorally-focused orgasms, while orgasms produced by stimulating the structures connected to the pelvic nerve branches feel more vaginal, uterine and anal. Playing with the structures and systems connected to the vagus nerve often produces a more whole-body and emotional orgasmic experience.

Here's the really big takeaway from this: *The more nerve pathways that you get activated, the more intense your pleasure will be.*

Lewd and Lascivious Ligaments

The *suspensory ligament* is a connective tissue cord that attaches to the glans and shaft of the clitoris. From the base of the clitoral shaft, it crosses up and over the pubic bone. The ligament then splits into two strands, with each attaching to the ligaments that hold the ovaries in place. It pulls the clitoral head up during sexual arousal, drawing it under the protective hood and sheltering it from over-stimulation.

The irony here is that many women, not yet having accessed the whole erectile network, depend on clitoral stimulation alone to get aroused and reach orgasm. You may want more direct clitoral stimulation, but Mother Nature is busy protecting the clitoral head from harm. (See Illustration: *The Transformations of Arousal* on page 123.)

Which gives us one more reason to activate the entire arousal network.

HOT TIPS FOR GUYS
A Tiny Target

Not only can the clitoral hood cover the head as a matter of course, but the head actually retracts under the hood as a woman gets more turned on. Since the head is quite small to begin with, usually about the size of a pea, the clit can be a very elusive target.

Here's some advice for you when you're a bit lost—ask for directions! I know it can be embarrassing, and it definitely violates the Guy Code, but we love it when you ask! Really, there's nothing sexier than a guy who makes it safe for us to tell him exactly what we like. It doesn't mean you're clueless, especially since what we like changes from day to day and moment to moment, depending on where we are in our cycle, how aroused we are, the time of day, and a multitude of other unpredictable factors. Trust me, there's no way anyone could get it right all the time without guidance.

Remember, the clit's sensitivity is extraordinary, so if you're doing something wonderful in the vicinity and then happen to do the same thing directly on the button, it can be a big ouch. Conversely, because it's so small, if you're doing something wonderful to it and you wander off target by a millimeter or two, you might cause her arousal to drop.

One last tip: when you find the perfect touch and the precise rhythm that's really getting us off, don't stop. Don't go faster or do it harder. Just keep on keeping on. Stay steady, consistent and relentless in doing that very right thing. We'll be very glad you did!

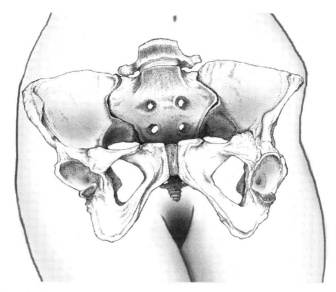

The Bony Bowl—Front View. *The pelvis inside the woman.*

The Bony Cradle

While often thought of as one piece, the pelvis is actually made up of three bones: the downward pointing triangle of the sacrum in the back, and the two wing-like iliac bones that form the front and sides of the bony bowl. The ilia meet in front with a cartilaginous seam to form the pubis, often called the pubic bone. The pelvic joints are normally capable of only a small amount of movement. Under the influence of the hormones of pregnancy, they become considerably more relaxed, which helps make it possible to open up enough to birth a baby.

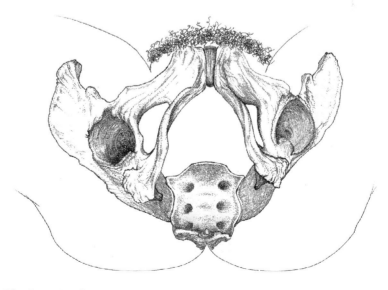

The Bony Bowl—Bottom View.

The Pulsing Pelvic Pump

The floor of your body is formed by a large group of muscles, collectively known as the pelvic floor. The *pelvic floor muscles* are arranged like a sling or hammock, attached in multiple places to the inner walls and bottom edges of the pelvis.

Since they go from the pubic bone in front to the tailbone (or coccyx) in back, they are also called the *pubococcygeus muscles*, mercifully shortened to the *PC muscles*.

"PC muscle" is the popular lay term for the pelvic floor muscles. It's a misnomer for two reasons. First, it confuses a part with the whole—the "PC muscle" technically refers only to the pubococcygeus muscles, not the entire pelvic floor muscle family. Second, the name implies there's just one big muscle when that's not the case. The pelvic floor muscles are actually a collection of muscles. One group is located toward the front of your body. These are the ones you use when you need to hold your pee in or push it out. Other pelvic floor muscles are located toward the rear. You use these to control your bowel movements. Plus, there's a whole group of muscles in between. The bladder, urethra, vagina, rectum and anus are surrounded by and pass through the multiple layers of pelvic floor muscles.

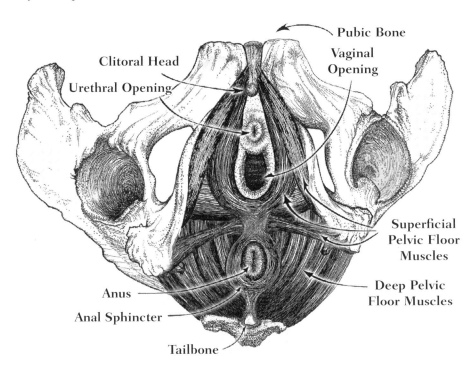

Pubic Bone

Vaginal Opening

Clitoral Head

Urethral Opening

Superficial Pelvic Floor Muscles

Deep Pelvic Floor Muscles

Anus

Anal Sphincter

Tailbone

The Pelvic Floor Muscles—*Bottom View. Shows the pelvic floor muscles in relation to the pelvic bones and urethral, vaginal and anal orifices.*

Some of the pelvic floor muscles are sphincter muscles, circular muscles that can open and close like a drawstring bag. The iris of your eye, with its ability to dilate and contract, is an example of a sphincter muscle. There are sphincters around the urethra, vagina, anus and rectum that help us open and close them.

"The function of muscle is to pull and not to push, except in the case of the genitals and the tongue."

LEONARDO DA VINCI

We also have circular sphincter muscles in our digestive tract, mouth, throat and eyes. All of these round muscles are neurologically connected and coordinated with each other. In consequence, what we do unto one will happen to others as well. This is why, when we want to relax and open our sex center, it helps to relax and open our mouth and throat.

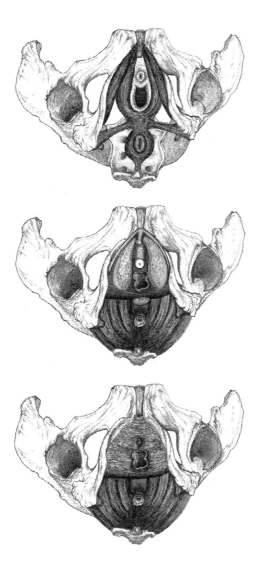

The Pelvic Floor Muscle Layers and Erectile Network Sandwich—Bottom View. On the top, you can see the top or superficial layer of muscles. The middle image shows what sits under the top layer—the erectile network, which rests on top of the deep muscle layer. The image on the bottom shows the deep layer. Note that the muscle group includes holes that allow for the urethral, vaginal and anal canals to pass through.

MASTERING YOUR INNER MUSCLES

Your inner pelvic muscles are one of the keys to turning yourself on. When you squeeze and release them, you're actually sexually playing with yourself without using your hands (or anyone else's). The pelvic floor muscle layers form a sandwich with your erectile network in the middle, so that moving these muscles directly stimulates your engorgeable tissue.

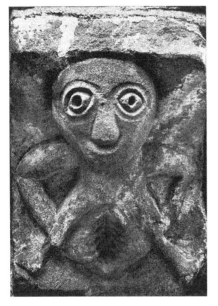

Ancient Irish Goddess—Sheila Na Gig

During orgasm, these muscles rapidly and rhythmically contract and release, sending waves of pleasure through the pelvis—and, if you're naturally lucky or have learned how, through the entire body.

You have both voluntary and involuntary control of these muscles. That is, you can let the muscles do their thing entirely on their own or, if you want to expand your experience, you can pump, pulsate and play with them as a unit or as separate sub-groups.

Whether you're a man or a woman, you can use the pelvic floor muscles to initiate your turn-on or add fuel to your sexual fire. Working them stimulates the nerves and increases the blood flow to your pelvis, which increases your engorgement and erection (or herection). The pelvic floor also acts like an energy trampoline, bouncing the sexual energy up into the rest of your body.

Keeping these muscles toned is important for general pelvic health throughout a woman's lifetime. They're also the muscles used to birth a baby. Strong, flexible and skilled muscles can facilitate efficient labor (a good thing), support the natural process (a very good thing), and even promote ecstatic birth (a great thing!). After childbirth, it is especially important to re-strengthen and tone these muscles. The pelvic floor muscles hold up the pelvic organs and keep gravity from having its way with a woman as she ages. For women with bladder control problems, a low or "dropped" uterus or "female" problems, or for anyone with constipation, strengthening these muscles can help enormously. And for women who wish to improve their sexual responsiveness, learning to work with these muscles is an all-important first step.

In fact, I'll take this further: getting in touch with your pelvic floor muscles is the foundation to becoming an erotic virtuoso. In the next section, I'll show you how to connect to and gain mastery of your powerful pelvic pump.

Glorious Glands

There are two sets of glands in the female genitalia.

Vestibular Glands

The *Bartholins glands* are a pair of grape-sized glands located at the bottom of the vaginal opening, with one on either side at five o'clock and seven o'clock, respectively. Since Bartholin didn't actually own a set of these glands himself, I prefer to call them the *vulvovaginal* or *vestibular glands*. They secrete a very small amount of fluid during arousal, probably to maintain a healthy vaginal ecology.*

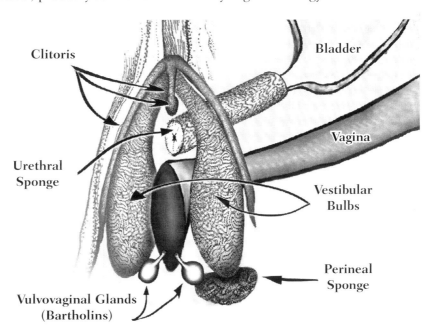

Vulvovaginal Glands—Bottom View. *You can see the two vulvovaginal (vestibular) glands, each with one small tubular duct, opening just inside the vaginal orifice.*

---

* Most medical professionals will say that these glands don't really have a function. It's a glib and inaccurate view. Surprisingly little research has been done on the glands, leaving medical professionals, no matter what they say, without much of a clue as to what they do or don't do. The prevailing medical attitude leads to questionable treatment strategies. Because the glands are viewed as unimportant, many doctors remove them if they cause recurrent problems. I suspect that, over time, we'll learn that these glands play an important role in supporting a healthy vaginal ecology. If that's the case, doing away with them as a nuisance is probably not the easy solution it seems to be. The paucity of data about the glands' function is striking and altogether too common in matters of women's health.

Paraurethral Glands

The second set of glands are called the *Skene's glands*, but since he didn't have any either, I prefer to call them the *paraurethral glands*. They're composed of a multitude of networks of tiny tubules, like the hair roots on a plant, which are enmeshed in the erectile tissue that sur-

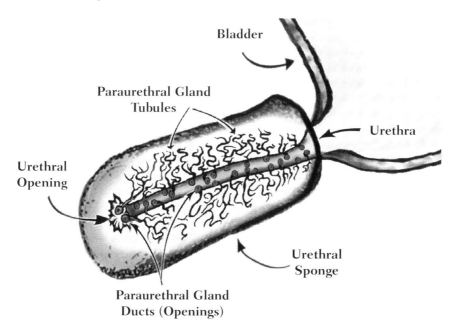

Paraurethral Glands in Urethral Sponge—A close-up of the urethral sponge, with the erectile tissue removed, reveals the multitude of tiny root-like tubules that make up the paraurethral glands. The tubules drain into ducts, creating multiple openings along the length of the urethra. Two slighter larger ducts are just inside the urethral orifice, with one small tubular duct opening just inside the vaginal orifice.

rounds and protects the urethra. This network of glandular tubules has about thirty ducts, or openings, along the length of the urethra as well as two main ducts that open just inside or outside the urethral orifice.

These glands are the source of female ejaculation, a clear watery fluid with a faint musky odor that can issue as a trickle, a small gush, or in great geysers of liquid. While "shejaculate" is most often expelled when a woman has an orgasm, it can also emerge during high-level arousal for some women.

All the ancient spiritual sexuality traditions considered female ejaculate to be a sacred medicine. Practitioners of ayurveda (the traditional medicine of India) and tantra called it *amrita*, meaning "the nectar of life." Taoist sexuality students and practitioners of traditional Chinese healing knew it as white moon flower medicine. In the tantric tradition, the fluid was collected in sacred ceremonies and either consumed for its holy and medicinal qualities, or directly expelled onto lucky recipients by priestesses as a blessing and healing practice.

Not all women who are orgasmic experience ejaculation. In fact, it seems to be a minority of women who do, and of the women who *do* gush, many don't do so every time. The most common time to squirt is after prolonged stimulation of the urethral sponge, often in the company of multiple orgasms.

There seems to be a small number of women who are what I call "natural ejaculators." They always do it and always have. For most women, however, this is a learned skill. If you're a woman who hasn't ejaculated yet, you can learn how. All women have the equipment and potential to squirt.

Embryologically, the urethral sponge is the same tissue that becomes the prostate in men. The ejaculate's make-up is similar to prostatic fluid, but much more watery. Although here, too, the medical establishment is behind the curve (or gush, as the case may be), I firmly believe that amrita contains multiple immune properties. It's produced by the paraurethral glands and designed to flood the urethra during and at the end of intercourse to protect the urinary system from infection, thus providing it with a third level of protection, in addition to the sponge's cushioning and narrowing functions.

I believe medical research will eventually confirm that both the vulvovaginal and paraurethral glands have important immune functions and that their presence is a necessary part of an intact and healthy vaginal environment. It makes sense since the glands are located at the two portals to the vagina and the urethra, just as other immune protection systems are located near entryways.*

Glorious Gushing Goddess

You may wonder why anyone would want to learn to squirt. The simple answer is—it feels wonderful. I have the good fortune to have learned to be able to gush, and when that happens, I feel like the goddess incarnate. When I gush on my partner, he too is blessed by this magical elixir. I highly recommend exploring this particular skill, which we'll be discussing in greater detail in Chapter Eleven.

---

* Think of the immune structures that protect our mouth and nose. We have tonsils, lymph nodes and adenoids. These are all immune-system components that protect us from nasty invaders. Why wouldn't women's lower orifices be similarly protected?

Last Butt Not Least

Our next stop on the anatomy tour is that much-maligned orifice, the *anus*. Yes, it's true: the asshole has gotten a bad rap. Of course, if you've ever had yours malfunction, you surely appreciate how wonderful this orifice is! For obvious reasons, though, the asshole is considered dirty and shameful.

THE GUIDED TOUR
Exploring the Garden of Anus

If you have never explored your own ass, there's no time like the present to begin. Start with a shower and make your rear end nice and clean. You can even do some exploring in the shower with a soapy finger!

If your play is post-shower, make sure to use some slippery lube: it makes for a much more agreeable experience. You may want to squat or kneel for easy access. Place your fingertip at the opening and see how it feels. Explore the edges. See if you can open your anus by breathing and bearing down slightly. Ease your finger in and feel around. You can also place your thumb in your pussy and find the fat place in the wall were your perineal sponge is located. Feel the thin place beyond that. Notice what you can do when you tighten and relax your anal sphincter muscles.

If you want to explore your anal pleasure potential, play with yourself in your usual favorite way, periodically adding ass stimulation, either at the opening or inside. Experiment with what feels good until you find what makes you go "oh!" There's a good chance something will.

You may want to buy a small or medium-sized butt plug and see if you like how that feels during your self-sex. Don't put anything up your ass that doesn't have a flanged base, otherwise it may go all the way in and be difficult to remove. That won't be fun (although it may give the folks in the emergency room a laugh). Only use toys that are specifically designed for ass play.

Personally, I believe this part of our anatomy merits a positive reframing. It should be appreciated not only for its important excretory functions, but for the enormous amount of pleasure that can be found in the sweet little rosebud of your butt. The anus is a vital and delightful part of your sexual equipment.

It's composed of a cone of muscle that forms two concentric sphincters, which, as noted earlier, are circular muscles that act like a drawstring or closure valve. The outer one is under voluntary control, while the inner sphincter is involuntary. The circle of anal muscles connects to the circular muscles of the vagina and forms a figure-eight, with the connection lying under the perineum and over the perineal sponge. (See Illustration: *Female Genitalia and Organs with Round Ligaments* on page 122 and *The Pelvic Floor Muscles* on page 130.)

The anus is lined with delicate mucosa that is full of highly sensitive nerve endings. In fact, the anus is second only to the rest of the genitalia in the number of nerve endings and therefore has exquisite pleasure potential.

> *"The word arse is as much god as the word face. It must be so, otherwise you cut off your god at the waist."*
>
> **D.H. LAWRENCE**

This isn't the only reason having something in your ass can feel so good. Remember that the perineal sponge is located in the triangular structure (called the *perineal body*) at the base of the thin wall between the anus and the vagina. As we've seen, it's made up of erectile tissue, meaning it, too, has the potential to feel really lovely. In addition, the major nerve bundles that innervate the back of the vagina also supply your rear equipment, branching into the thin wall between the canals.

The anus is the last section of the gastro-intestinal tract. Just before the anus is the rectum, where your poop rests until it's ready to move down, giving you that "I need to go *now*" sensation, which you respond to by heading for the toilet. What this means is that most of the time, your feces aren't hanging out in your anus. The anus is a transit passageway and, in this sense, not unlike the urethra.

This isn't to suggest the anus is squeaky-clean. It's not. Anything that's come in contact with or been inside your ass should be considered contaminated by butt-microbes and unsuitable for pussy play.

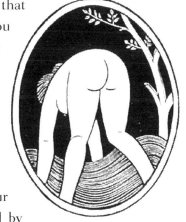

ERIC GILL

It's also the case, though, that the, er, brown-ness of the anal experience is typically quite modest. Put it this way: most ass play isn't full of shit.

Owner's Manual
Sexual Segregation

It's important to be conscious of what goes where, since you don't want the finger or toy (or whatever) that's been touching your ass to then be in contact with your yoni. Bacteria from your rear need to stay there. If they get in your vagina or urethra, you can get a nasty infection. Ass play is great, but it needs to be combined with strict segregation and great sexual hygiene.

. . . .

HOT TIPS FOR GUYS
Getting In the Garden

Ah, the taboo desire . . . to get into her nether hole! Well, gentlemen, let me suggest something to you. You, too, have an asshole, and there's no better way to learn to play with hers than by playing with your own. Play with it and you'll very quickly learn how to make her ass (and yours!) very happy.

While you're at it, you might also suggest to her that she do some personal ass-play, too. After all, there's nothing like learning together!

One thing will become immediately clear to you when you start playing with yourself. The ass is very yin. It needs to be wooed open, and this requires time and gentleness. You can't hurry ass-play.

Remember these three words with regard to butt play: *slow, conscious*, and *well-lubed*. (Okay, maybe it's four words.)

For this to be the great fun it can be, you will also need to communicate carefully and often. Before you begin, check in about her boundaries and desires in this department, and don't under any circumstances transgress her limits. Pressure will get you nowhere except, maybe, shown the door. Patience, understanding, caring and communication, plus slowly opening her pleasure pathways, will get you to your goal.

Once she's ready to explore ass play, get her in a state of high arousal. Along with plenty of stimulation to her clit, add gentle well-lubed attention to the outside of her anal opening. If she likes that and gives the go-ahead, gently slide your slippery finger in a bit, or alternatively use a butt toy.

Once she feels comfortable with something small, you may find her eager to try your cock. This may not happen during your first session or, for that matter, your tenth. Don't rush or pressure her. It's important to be patient. It's an activity she may come to love over time.

Once she's ready to try your penis, start off by getting her really hot. As before, use your finger or a butt toy to relax and warm up her anus. Continue to stimulate her clitoris throughout your ass exploration, either by doing it yourself or having her do it. Once she's wild and willing, remove the small-ish object you've been warming her up with and very slowly, with frequent stops and check-ins, slide your cock into her ass.

(We'll pause to imagine the pleasure.)

And, oh yes, did I mention *slowly*? Let me say it again. She needs to open up around you, so proceed ultra-deliberately, pausing after each incremental insertion for her to breathe and relax around you. Remind her to dilate, relax, breathe and make opening sounds. Go at her pace, stop when she says to, and withdraw immediately if she requests it. If you gain her ass's trust, it will open for you. Once she gets aroused and loosens up around you, that's the time to begin more active movements. Again, ramp it up slowly. If you take the time she needs, you can both enjoy the intensity and wild pleasure of being total butt-sluts.

And remember, once anything (finger, toy, cock, or whatever) has visited the butt, it can't go play in the pussy until it's been thoroughly washed with soap and water.

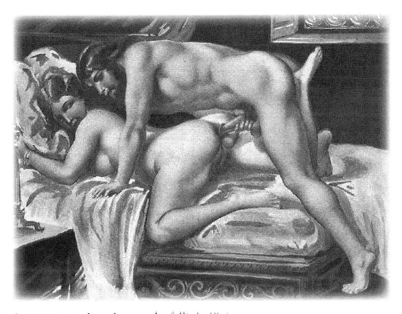

Anonymous—*based on work of Giulo Pipi*

CHAPTER EIGHT

Circuits and Cycles, Conduits and Connections

*"There are only two ways to live your life.
One is as though nothing is a miracle.
The other is as though everything is a miracle."*

ALBERT EINSTEIN

Titillation

IN THIS CHAPTER, WE CONSIDER WOMEN'S anatomy of arousal from a higher-level, whole-system perspective. But before we explore these circuits and connections, we need to take one more anatomical expedition and travel north to the breasts. Any discussion of female anatomy would be woefully lacking without a detour to this titillating territory.

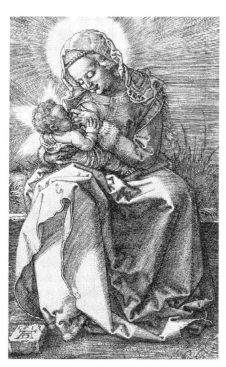

ALBRECHT DÜRER—*Madonna Nursing*

The female *breast* is a marvelous, multi-function structure. First and foremost, the mammary glands are perfectly designed to nurture a new human being by providing love, physical contact, stimulation, regulation of bodily systems and rhythms, and ideal nutrition. It is also a luscious erogenous zone, conveniently hard-wired by nerves and hormones into both the brain and the uterus.

All breasts are composed of fatty tissue that surrounds a series of glandular tubules. In the approximate center of the breast is the circular darker areola, each surmounted by a (usually) raised nipple. Under the areola, the small glandular tubules swell and form the milk sinuses, which then feed into tiny tubes with many minute openings in the nipple. Nipples and areolae are composed of a healthy amount of erectile tissue, which accounts for their capacity to sit up and take notice, whether it's due to a suckling infant, an attentive partner or a cool breeze.

Women have a delightful variety of breast sizes. Big or small, the magnitude of the breast has absolutely nothing to do with its capacity to produce milk or receive pleasure. Here, too, size doesn't matter. All breasts contain the same amount of milk-producing tissue, just as we all have the same number of ribs or teeth. The variation in breast size is mere window dressing. The differences evolved over time in response to social and sexual selection pressure. Big breasts advertise fertility and are one of nature's strategies for attracting mates.

After prepping by the hormones of pregnancy, breast-feeding is a simple supply-and-demand system, with the breasts making as much milk as the baby (or babies) require for as long as needed. Under the areola lie nerve receptors that respond to the mechanical stimulation of suckling by making milk. It's that simple: more sucking makes more mamma juice.

While the relatively rugged areolae are designed to take the intense vacuum suction of a baby's mouth, the extremely delicate nipple is just the opposite. During nursing, the sensitive nipple is supposed to be drawn deeply into the baby's mouth and shouldn't actually get sucked or

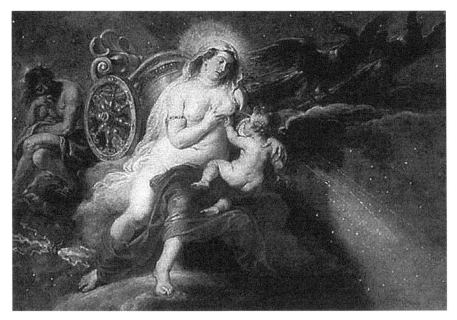

Peter Paul Rubens—*The Milky Way, c. 1600*

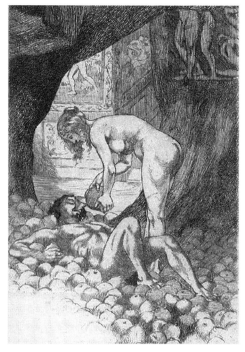

MARTIN VAN MAELE—*Francion*

"I have seen the ads for the Wonder Bra. Is that really a problem in this country? Men not paying enough attention to women's breasts?"

HUGH GRANT

rubbed at all. In fact, if the baby is sucking on the nipple, instead of the areola, it will hurt, cueing mom that the baby isn't properly latched on.

The breast itself contains fat and glands covered by delicate skin. The glands respond to women's hormonal rhythms and can undergo dramatic changes in size, texture and sensitivity during the menstrual cycle, as well as during pregnancy, breast-feeding and menopause.

Our cultural fixation on breasts has laid a heavy energetic and emotional charge on them. Breasts are beautiful, but don't deserve the extreme reactions they elicit, from implant madness and adolescent ogling to burying them under layers of loose clothing or decrying them as profane.

Beyond this cultural "boobhaha," breasts offer wonderful learning opportunities. They are a great starting point for women to love their body as it is. Men can learn to appreciate breasts without ignoring their owners while also supporting women to be okay with their breasts and bodies, whatever their size and shape. Hopefully we can also get past our widespread fear of nipples and support breast-feeding as the norm it should be.*

---

* Breast-feeding promotes health and well-being by reducing the incidence of every known disease throughout the life span. It protects against everything from colic to Alzheimer's, from allergies to auto-immune disease, and from obesity to addiction while also increasing intelligence and psychological health. Nothing produced in a factory comes close to this mammary miracle food.

HOT TIPS FOR GUYS
Let's Look at Breasts

Hmm ... well, guys, maybe your hot tip should be to *not* look at the breasts, just this once!

But seriously, men, the breasts need to be treated expertly, too.

First, don't head there before it's time. Remember what I said earlier about playing with the non-erogenous zones before heading toward hotter territory? I know how alluring the breasts can be. Still, don't fixate on them. You'll have plenty of time to play with them when she's good and ready. Check in with her if you're not sure.

Second, remember—babies suck ferociously on areolae, not nipples. There's a lesson to be learned from this. The areola is designed to respond to strong, rhythmic stimulation and can often be handled quite firmly with excellent results. You need to handle the sensitive nipples with great care, though. Don't play rough with them unless she asks for it.

It's also important to take into account the woman's cycle, as her mammary glands respond to her hormonal dances as well as her arousal level. Different times of the month—and differing levels of arousal— mean different modes of handling.

(Yes, women are complicated.)

Clit Notes Summary of Women's Anatomy of Arousal

In the preceding chapters, we conducted a part-by-part tour of the female genitalia, including the erectile network. Before proceeding to the next part of our discussion, which takes a system-level look at women's sexual anatomy, let's review what we've learned so far.

Women's erectile network is made up of the interconnected but separate structures of the clitoris, vestibular bulbs and two sponges. The clitoris is composed of three parts, the head, the shaft and the legs. The paired vestibular bulbs form fat parentheses around the vaginal opening, lying under the lips. The urethral sponge is the tubular cylinder of erectile tissue that surrounds the urethra and lies above the roof of the vagina. The perineal sponge is a pad of erectile tissue that sits under the vaginal floor, in the wall between the vaginal and anal canals.

The inner labia also include some loosely distributed erectile tissue. The anal sphincter probably does as well. And erectile tissue isn't limited to your nether regions. Nipples and areolae are full of it, as their perky responsiveness demonstrates. We also have it in our lips, earlobes and the flaring opening of our nostrils—the better to see, smell and taste you with, as any bad wolf knows!

THE AROUSAL ARRANGEMENTS

While all erectile tissue is essentially the same, the energy, arrangement and responses of the female arousal apparatus are strikingly different from the male's.

First, women can get aroused and be orgasmic with only part of the network activated. Unlike the all-or-nothing instrument of the penis, the female arousal network consists of many instruments. When one or two instruments are playing, the results are good—very good, sometimes! But women's arousal and orgasmic experiences depend on which areas of their network have been ignored or stimulated so when the entire erectile orchestra is playing, the quality of the music rises to an entirely new and ecstatically enchanting level. This is no mere happenstance— the structures are connected at multiple levels and designed to play well together. It's one of Mother Nature's strategies for ensuring that reproduction is an activity women will want to do eagerly and often.

Second, women's capacity for multiple orgasms appears to be related to the microscopic details of her erectile network. In women's erectile capillaries, even with orgasm, some valves open and others stay closed, meaning that some herection remains. While the path to female orgasm may be more elusive than the one for men to begin with, once it's discovered, the next step into multi-orgasmic capability is often an easy journey to make.

Third, unlike men, women generally do not like having their erectile structures stimulated until they are already at least partly engorged. Premature stimulation is irritating and can actually decrease arousal. This is because yin sexual energy moves from the outside to the center. Yin arousal energy needs some time to accumulate in the genitals before direct contact is appreciated. This stands in stark contrast to how yang energy starts—right smack dab in the sex center. That's why core yang folk (or anyone in a yang mood) typically respond eagerly to direct genital stimulation at the onset of interactions . . . or as soon as possible.

A Single, Complex, Integrated System

Here's the straightforward (and elegant) reality: women's sexual and reproductive structures and systems are one connected, coordinated, integrated arrangement. Sex, pregnancy, birth, orgasm, breast-feeding, bleeding (and not bleeding)—all participate in the same grand system. Science tends to break systems down into their components, in the process often overlooking the fact that the whole is much greater than the sum of the parts. It's an approach that has its virtues, but misses the forest for the trees. While the female sexual system does depend on the contributions of muscles, hormones, nerves, psyche, energy, neurochemistry and more, it's not just a compilation of parts. It's a unified, brilliantly designed system, and we're missing something important if we don't see it in that light.

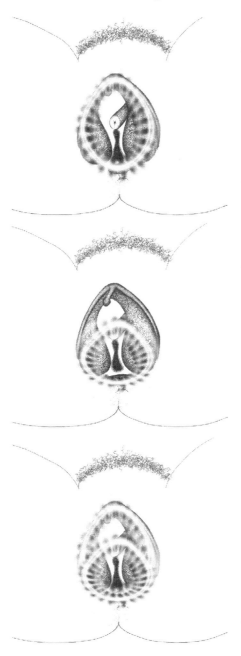

INTERTWINING CIRCUITS

We'll begin by returning to women's erectile network, which includes the three-part clitoris, the vestibular bulbs, and the two sponges. These are not just separate, one-off ways to get off: they were designed to work together as a system. The erectile network forms two interwoven circuits. One forms the cuff around the vaginal opening, while the second overlaps the cuff and includes the whole clitoris.

When both erectile circuits are engaged and engorged, stimulation and penetration feel marvelous. Without all the structures pleasured and puffed, insertion and thrusting are not nearly so arousing and may be downright uncomfortable.

The Erectile Circuits—*The adjacent erectile structures create linked circuits. One ring surrounds the entrance of the vagina, connecting the side walls, floor and roof. A second circuit is formed that includes the entire clitoris. The two circuits overlap and intertwine.*

ERECTILE EXPANSION—
THE NETWORK AT PLAY

Let's take a closer look at what happens when the entire arousal orchestra is engaged. At high turn-on, the mind is in an altered state, utterly absorbed in the erotic experience. The body is awash with feel-good chemicals. Muscles tighten, the breath comes fast and deep, the heart pounds and senses focus on pleasure. Blood flow has dramatically increased to the erogenous areas. Nipples perk, lips swell, the nostrils flare and the pelvic region is flooded. Nerves snap to attention and electric energy buzzes through the sexual circuits.

In the genital arena, the entire clitoris enlarges, becoming increasingly and exquisitely sensitive to the movement of the surrounding tissues—lips, mons, hood and the muscles on top and underneath. The vestibular bulbs go from being a small side note to a seriously swollen presence, pressing in on the vaginal orifice from either side. The vagina is both snugger and more expandable due to the erectile tissue's clever capacity to swell and stretch.

The Transformation of the Erectile Network—When stimulated, the erectile network undergoes impressive changes as it becomes tumescent. Top: Not engorged. Middle: Medium arousal and engorgement. Bottom: Fully engorged.

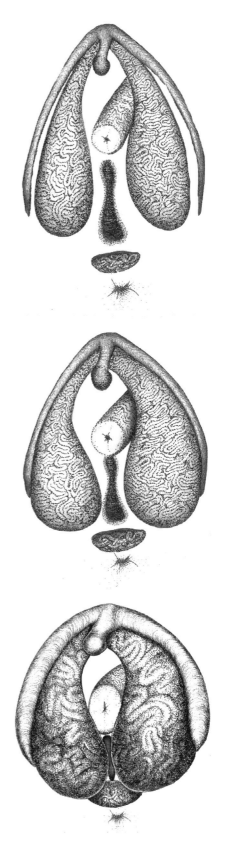

THE BLOOMING VULVA

The vulva blooms open like a fleshy, fertile flower. For many women, the head of the clitoris won't be visible (though yours may be), but for all women, it will be swollen whether or not it's hidden beneath its hood. The head and shaft widen, expanding the tent of tissue above them. Beneath their sheath of muscle, the clitoral legs also swell, interacting pleasurably with the interlacing muscles of the pelvic floor. The *bulbo-cavernosus*, the large sphincter muscle that encircles the vaginal orifice, is stretched and widened by the tumescent bulbs beneath.

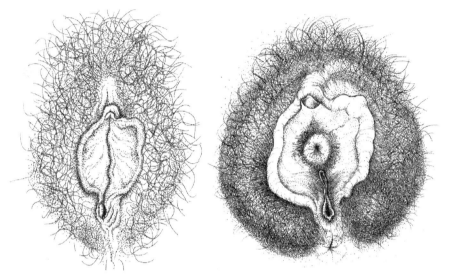

The Transformation of the Vulva—*The enlargement of the erectile network visibly distends the entire vulva. Left: The vulva at rest. Right: The dramatic blooming of the vulva is evident with full engorgement of the entire erectile network.*

The outer labia are pushed open by the fattened bulbs, exposing more of the usually hidden intimate areas. The inner labia swell, darkening delightfully. The end of the urethral sponge is puffed—sitting just at the top of the vaginal opening, or perhaps a bit inside—to the point where the outer end is visible from the vestibule; you can see the raised circular cushion around the urethral opening. Any pussy penetration at this point will pull the outer pad of the urethral sponge along with it during in-and-out action.

THE INNER ORCHESTRA

The same muscle that surrounds the vaginal orifice and covers the distended bulbs also provides the place of attachment for the round ligaments. As these ropy muscles contract, they tug the uterus forward and up. The perineal sponge in the anal-vaginal wall expands, pressing into both canals. The roof of the vagina bulges dramatically down as the urethral sponge swells along its entire length. The increased circulation causes the walls of the pussy to "sweat," producing their slick lubrication. The back of the vaginal vault is opened as the cervix is drawn upward, exposing the locations on either side in the back where the nerves bundles enter.

As arousal energy builds, the tension mounts as the pussy puffs and circuits swell. Like a pumped-up blood-pressure cuff, the genital cuff is inflated and squeezing snugly. When her herection is complete, the whole circuit of erectile expansion is evident.

During orgasm, the orchestra pulses in a variety of rhythms—the muscles happily and quickly quivering, the clitoris pulsing, sponges squeezing and squirting, the uterus bopping up and down while the brain goes on holiday and the tide pounds in pleasure. Sex and the single clit is a good thing: sex and the integrated erectile circuits—in other words, sex at the system level—is much better!

And why stop there? Sex that integrates the four main aspects of our being—body, mind, heart and spirit—is the best of all.

Now that we've looked at the circuits on the physical level, let's take a look at the big evolutionary picture.

SEX, FERTILITY, AND BIRTH—ONE ECSTATIC SYSTEM

In humans, sex and reproduction, love and lust, and care and connection all overlap and interconnect. It makes evolutionary sense that this is so. While it's certainly possible to have unconnected, uncaring sex, we are definitely hard-wired for connection.

This is especially true for women, for whom sex is a high-risk activity. Female humans have limited reproductive opportunities, unlike males with their unending supply of sperm. Pregnancy and child-rearing are activities that require an enormous amount of time and energy. Since it takes human babies many years to become independent, and since two can raise a family

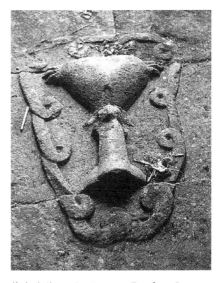

Sukah Temple, Karang Pandan, Java

more easily than one, having sex with someone you are emotionally bonded to tends to be a successful reproductive strategy.

There are not two separate systems, one for pleasure and one for reproduction. It's all one integrated, multi-purpose arrangement. As we've already discussed, there are hardwired physical, energetic and emotional circuits connecting the various erectile matrix components with each other, the uterus with the vaginal opening, and the breasts with the uterus.

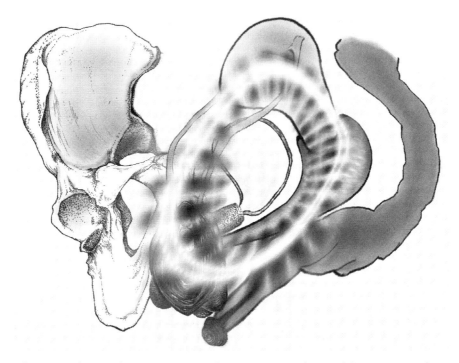

The Sex and Reproduction Circuit—*The impressive and powerful movements of the uterus during arousal and orgasm function to support and maximize fertility. A physical and energetic circuit runs from the vaginal opening in and along the canal, up through the uterus, up along the round ligaments, over the pubic bone and back to the vaginal opening.*

Our culture tends to see birth and sex as unrelated activities. Not that people don't understand that sex is what gets the baby started, but the subsequent processes—pregnancy, birth and breast-feeding—are generally seen as maternal, not sexual. This is a false dichotomy. The fact is that arousal and labor are very similar, and so are orgasm and birth. While it's true that sex is intensely pleasurable and birth is wildly intense (and often intensely painful), both are consuming, extraordinary and powerful processes that are similar by evolutionary design, and not by coincidence.

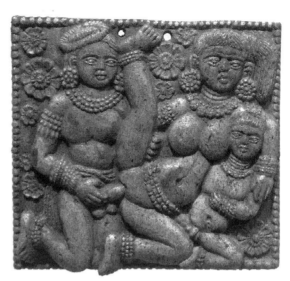

Sunga period, 1st century BCE

Sex and giving birth are not just two ends of a journey: they are the same journey, an intimately connected system that follows a primal evolutionary template.

Evolutionary design conservatively uses the same equipment, energy and biochemical tides in both the sex and birth experiences. Both journeys also involve similarly altered states of consciousness, with the kindred trance states choreographed by the same chemistry:

- Oxytocin is a key player in the dance as it stimulates the contractions of labor, breast-feeding and orgasm. This so-called "love hormone" inspires attachment and mothering, be it to your beloved baby or your sweet soulmate.

- The falling-in-love hormone, phenylethylamine, or PEA, supports the magic of new baby bonding as well as the overwhelming passion of new lovers.

- Endorphins, our natural opiates, flood women whether they're in the throes of passion or labor.

- Dimethyltryptamine, or DMT, dubbed the "god chemical" because of its association with transcendent experiences when used as a recreational drug, is released by the pineal gland in small bursts during regular orgasm, in sustained flow with expanded orgasm, and in labor, peaking at birth.

Both the first stage of labor and the process of arousal are yin—they involve surrender, release and opening. Each requires a person to go with the flow, turn inwards and become entranced. Both orgasm and the decidedly more yang propulsive second part of labor involve adrenalin-mediated action.

Also, either process can get derailed by the same antagonists—fear, anxiety and the inability to trust and to open. Yet another antagonist for both is stimulation of the analytical neocortical brain, which can cause either process to stall.

Despite our generalized cultural anxiety, labor and birth have the potential to be powerful, transformative and even ecstatic experiences. Some women actually have orgasms during the birthing process!

As a practical matter, it's useful to keep the parallels between sex and birth in mind. As a midwife with over two decades' experience birthing babies, I can say with certainty that, to have the best possible birth experience, you should choose your birth place the same way you'd select a place to make love—where you'll feel safe, private and undisturbed. Surround yourself with trustworthy allies and people who have faith in the innate wisdom of the natural birth process. Only when a woman feels secure can she open to the powerful tides of arousal or labor and release into orgasm, birth or ideally orgasmic birth in a flood tide of pleasure, wonder and love.

Breast-feeding is also part of women's sexual experience, as it's designed to be a pleasurable and even ecstatic lovefest between the sacred and intertwined dyad of mama and baby. The hormones of in-loveness and bonding are there to help us survive the exhausting demands of parenting

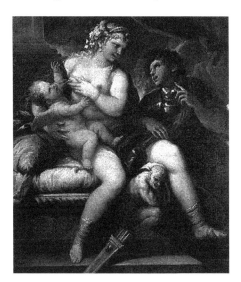

LUCA GIORDANO—*Venus, Cupid and Mars*

"No one who has seen a baby sinking back satiated from the breast and falling asleep with flushed cheeks and a blissful smile can escape the reflection that this picture persists as a prototype of the expression of sexual satisfaction in later life."

SIGMUND FREUD

and ensure that we nurture our offspring instead of ignoring or abandoning them, as we'd surely do if we didn't love them madly.

All the aspects of the journey—cycles, fertility, pregnancy, arousal, orgasm, birth and breast-feeding—are part of the integral whole that is female sexuality.

It is one of the tragedies of our culture that we've severed pregnancy, birth and breast-feeding from their messy, earthy, embodied sexual roots. To fully appreciate female sexuality, we must remember (and re-member) these connections, which hold true at a primordial level whether the woman in question chooses (or is able) to reproduce or not.

Beyond that, we must also bear in mind that the integral nature of female sexuality does not begin and end with the body. The emotions are involved, too. There are not separate processes for love and lust. All these circuits are connected to and by your big old sexy brain.

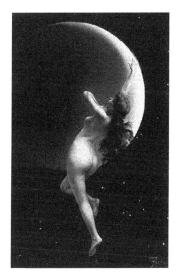

Luis Ricardo Falero—
The Moon Nymph, 1896

The Magic of the Menstrual Moon—The Waxing and Waning Cycle

Everyone, both men and women, can benefit from having a usable understanding of the female fertility cycle. If you want to know about the elaborately choreographed dance of the hormones, there are plenty of sources. Let's skip over that and look at the cycle from an energetic point of view. The physiological and psychological dynamics underlying women's menstrual cycle provide elegant insights into how sex, reproduction and the emotions are part of a single, integrated system.

Women's fertility cycle used to be attuned to the moon's rhythm of twenty-eight to twenty-nine days. All women in a tribe or family who weren't pregnant or menopausal bled at the same time. In primal cultures, it continues to be the case that women bleed during the dark moon and ovulate at the full. Due to artificial lighting and other factors, most civilized women have lost that attunement. However, menstrual synchronization sometimes still occurs, as women who have lived together know.

Like the moon, the monthly menstrual cycle waxes and then wanes. The first half of the cycle begins with the first day of bleeding (Day One) and extends through ovulation. This is the waxing part, much like the moon that gets bigger and brighter each night.

Ovulation is the turning point. In primal cultures, which is to say in cultures unaffected by artificial technological interference, this occurs with the full moon—women are likeliest to get pregnant when the moon is at its roundest. Once the full moon and ovulation are past, the second (or waning) half of the cycle begins and continues until the beginning of the next period.

The first part of the cycle lasting from menses to egg is variable in length. It usually lasts between twelve and sixteen days, although this can fluctuate wildly from woman to woman and for individual women, too. (This is one of the reasons it's difficult to predict when a woman is fertile, since the timing of ovulation can vary considerably.)

The second part of the cycle, from ovulation until the next period, is fixed. It's almost always exactly fourteen days for all women.

THE WEEKLY WEATHER REPORT

To really understand the energetics of the fertility cycle, it is important to remember the evolutionary template is geared towards reproduction. We currently have the privilege of utilizing modern methods to prevent conception, so cycles and fertility can be turned towards things other than babies. Still, a woman's monthly journey has an emotional and erotic rhythm that is laid down by primal, universal reproductive impulses and operates independently of whether, as a modern, self-aware adult, she does or doesn't have or want to have a baby.

WEEK ONE: THE BLEEDING TIME. During the first week of the cycle, which can be characterized as the bleeding time, the moon is shadowed and the night is very dark.* Bleeding means that you have not created a new life with your previous egg, and you (or rather that primal, born-to-breed part of you) now release that hope. The blood flows, as do the emotions. Menstruation is a time of letting go, of releasing, of death preparing for rebirth. The energy is turned in, poised, quiet and insightful. There is an element of grieving as you release what hasn't worked and mourn the little deaths and losses of your life. You crave comfort and your tears may flow easily as you discharge and let loose.

---

* Women's periods typically range from three to eight days.

In traditional cultures, this was a time of deep, expansive spiritual work. All the bleeding women would gather in a special place and do ritual for the healing of the world, fertility of the earth, and planetary visioning. They would be exempt from their normal duties and responsibilities while they did the sacred journeying that only blood magic could catalyze.

For modern women, the period of bleeding can be a great time to claim space for yourself or to follow the lead of primal people and gather with other women. Energetically, this is when it makes the most sense to take a break from serving and caring for others. It also lends itself to letting go of the old. This is when you can allow your flow to carry off with it everything you no longer need and release what no longer serves you.

WEEK TWO: WAXING TOWARDS FULLNESS. After your period ends, you move into the time of optimism and vigor. As the moon grows bigger and brighter each night, waxing towards full, so do women. This is the upward and outward phase of the cycle as each day brings you closer to ovulation. Your vitality and energy levels increase, as does your libido. Your energy and vision are directed outwards: you are seeking that special spark of attraction, intuitively knowing the time is approaching when you can create new life (regardless of your actual desire to make a baby).

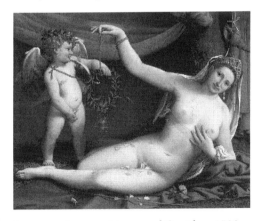

LORENZO LOTTO—*Venus and Cupid, c. 1500*

Week Two is when women are most inclined to be social, outgoing and extroverted. Although humans have what's called occult or hidden ovulation, this doesn't keep women from sending, and men from receiving, a wide variety of subtle signals about breeding status. Scientific studies have established that Week Two is when women are most likely to dress in sexy skimpy clothes, when they're most likely to be talked to and touched by men in casual settings, and when men find them most attractive. This is also a time of peak intelligence for women and the time we do best on tests of all kinds.

Week Two is the period leading up to peak fertility on the actual day of egg release, though women can get pregnant for five days prior to ovulation. (This is because, as we saw earlier, a woman's body can keep sperm alive for up to five days in "sperm hotels," tiny glandular pockets just inside the cervix.) During Week Two, the vagina is at its most robust; it is especially well-lubricated and ready for action. The cervix adds a flow of slick and slippery stuff, charmingly called fertile mucus, that makes everything—and not just sperm!—slide delightfully.

Thus we have yet another example of our clever evolutionary design. We just happen to want to have sex the most, and are most apt to find a mate, during that time of the month when we're likeliest to make a baby. Libido peaks on the day of ovulation. Women project the energy of maximum fertility. We shine like the full moon, bright and glorious.

> *"Where do babies come from? Don't bother asking adults.*
> *They lie like pigs. However, diligent independent research*
> *and hours of playground consultation have yielded*
> *fruitful, if tentative, results. There are several theories.*
> *Near as we can figure out, it has something to do with*
> *acting ridiculous in the dark."*
>
> *Bongo, From "Childhood Is Hell"*
> *by* MATT GROENING

WEEK THREE: THE WANING MOON. The egg has come, provided a brief opportunity for conception and now, if unfertilized, passes. With the death of the egg, everything pivots and the energy that was going up and out starts heading down and in. Each new day is characterized by a waning of vitality and libido.

WEEK FOUR: IT'S GETTING DARKER. Along with the shrinking moon, the energy continues to diminish. A woman's vision and thoughts turn inwards, often revealing issues that weren't evident in the first three weeks of the cycle. What is commonly thought of as bitchiness is really women looking at the deep issues and relationships in their lives with the intense gaze of the inner eye and questioning what isn't working.

This is a fragile time for the vagina—and the rest of us, too. It's when we're likeliest to feel depressed, fatigued and uninterested in sex. Rather than go out, we would rather stay in and think (or brood, as the case may be).* It's also when women are most prone to get vaginal infections and other types of illness.

---

* Etymologically, the word "brood" is related to the word breed.

This is a time to give yourself lots of self-love. It's also a time to honor this part of your cycle by creating a low-stress atmosphere of comfort and rest. Ideally, your intimate partners will be understanding of the special challenges this time of the month poses, and treat you with extra tenderness and love.

Just because Week Four is when women are most likely to identify relationship issues and life challenges doesn't make it the best time to try to solve them. Taking action can overload an already burdened system. It is a time for gentle treatment, not bold action.

As we go more deeply into Week Four, the nights keep getting darker, until the relief and release of bleeding time blessedly arrives.

And then this dance—this choreography of all that's primal (blood and birth, desire and retreat, sex and death), this dance of a woman's most eternal qualities, this integral rhythm which is danced by the light of the moon—all begins again.

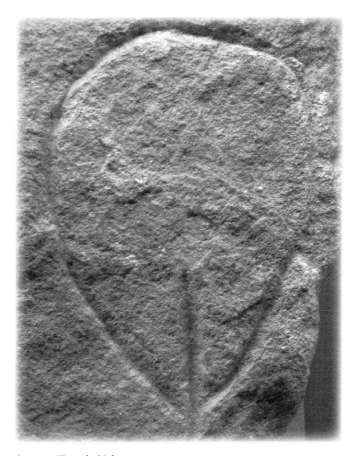

Ancient Temple Vulva

Becoming an
Erotic Virtuoso

*"We cannot teach people anything; we can only
help them discover it within themselves."*

—GALILEO GALILEI

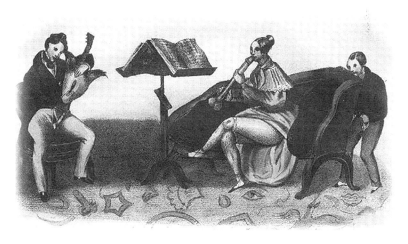

Achille Deveria—*Musicians, 1857*

CHAPTER NINE

Head Games and Heart-Ons

It's Your Turn

IN SECTION ONE, I PROVIDED FRAMEWORKS for better understanding sexuality in general, your sexuality specifically and sexuality in our culture. In Section Two, we got down to anatomical specifics. And now, in Section Three, it's time to transform what you've learned into erotic virtuosity.

In this section, I'll be discussing four sets of tools, one for each core aspect of our being: mind, heart, body and spirit. We'll also be exploring working with energy and what I call "smart slut tricks—advanced techniques for giving yourself and your partner fabulous pleasure. (As discussed later, I use "slut" in a positive sense to mean anyone who absolutely loves sex.)

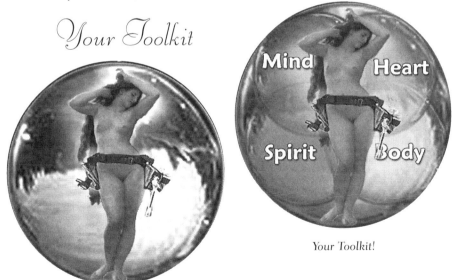

Your Toolkit?

Your Toolkit!

In this chapter, we'll look at mind and heart tools; in Chapter Ten, we'll turn our attention to body and spirit skills; and in Chapter Eleven, our focus will be on energy and sluttery.

While I don't give each major skill set equal time, this doesn't mean they're not equally important. How much coverage each gets has been dictated by one consideration only: how much information I thought needed to be conveyed to really get you going on your journey of erotic mastery.*

Each of the four realms has its own set of learnable skills. You can think of them in different ways:

- As a tool like a hammer or an instrument like a piano

- As the skill to use the tool—not the hammer itself, but the ability to wield it with expertise or to play your piano skillfully

- Or, you can scale the image up to the next level and picture your toolkit as a symphony orchestra. In other words, you are simultaneously each instrument, each individual musician and the conductor coordinating it all. (It's a useful way to look at it if you don't mind having multiple personality disorder.)

It's important to remember that, just as the map is not the territory, the metaphor is not the thing. Needless to say, you're a whole lot more than a tool or an instrument. You're really more like an athlete, and the instrument you're learning to play is . . . *yourself*. Through training and practice, it—in other words, *you*—can become more and more finely tuned.

Practice—it's an interesting word. It means doing something repeatedly until you get good at it ("I'm going to practice the guitar"), and it also means something you make a deep commitment to ("I have a spiritual practice"). My advice to you? Embrace both! You're much likelier to become an erotic virtuoso if you make a practice of practice.

> *"The sexual embrace can only be compared with music and with prayer."*
>
> MARCUS AURELIUS
> *(Roman emperor, AD 121–180)*

Framing Your Erotic Learning Journey

Learning is its own art form. Let's look at some guiding principles that can help you get the most out of your learning journey.

---

* I also don't give equal time to every sub-skill. Again, please don't read this to mean they are unequally important. The length of these sections is strictly a function of how much I felt I needed to say to provide you with foundational skills.

Our focus in this book is on *solo tools and skills*. Since your sexuality is rooted in your relationship with yourself, it makes sense to start by focusing not on what you do with partners, but on what you do with . . . *you*. After all, at the end of the day, it's not your lover who's responsible for your pleasure: it's you. Before you can make fabulous music with someone else, you need to master your own instrument.

We use the same skills to play with others that we use to play with ourselves, so what you're learning now can be put to good use later in partner play. The tools you'll be learning here have two levels—how you use them solo, and how you use them with a partner. Second-level relationship skills or "relationskills" are generally more complex and advanced than the solo skills that are the focus of this book.

Your Wholistic Sexuality Tools: Levels of Learning and Skill

The Wholistic Sexuality curriculum has three distinct levels. You might think of it as having undergraduate and master's levels, followed by a Ph.D.

LEVEL ONE consists of solo skills. These are tools that support self-connection and erotic encounters with yourself:

- Your foundational sexual skill set involves learning how to use your body, mind, spirit and heart tools. This is the toolkit you need to play your own instrument.

- All of your advanced skills are built on this foundation, whether you use the tools with yourself or with others.

- Solo skills range from the basic (for instance, orgasmic proficiency) to the considerably more advanced (orgasmic abundance).

LEVEL TWO focuses on basic relation skills (partner skills):

- This skill set uses your basic Level One toolkit in expanded ways.

- They involve learning to create connection and how to play duets with partners.

LEVEL THREE teaches advanced partner skills. It brings in new skills above and beyond your basic toolkit. When you've mastered the advanced relationskills of Level Three, you'll have your Ph.D. in erotic virtuosity and know how to play really, really nicely (and naughtily) with others!

PRACTICE MAKES ACCESS

Learning sex skills is no different from learning anything else that requires mental and muscle memory. Whatever you're learning becomes easier over time as the patterns become embedded in our bodies and brains. It's not unlike learning to drive a car. At first, it can seem impossibly complicated. How can one possibly steer, work the pedals, pay attention to the road and watch out for other cars, all while trying to navigate and not kill anyone? Over time, it gets easier until it eventually becomes something we can do automatically.

> *"We are what we repeatedly do. Excellence, then, is not an act, but a habit."*
>
> **ARISTOTLE**

Solo sex is no different. Just as you became a skilled auto driver, you can become an expert driver of your autoerotic self.

Start with what's easy and stretch from there into more challenging territory, allowing your skills sets to build on each other. Begin by practicing the basics over and over again. Eventually, you'll become adept at these skills and the learning will become embodied. This will then serve as your foundation as you progress to more advanced skills.

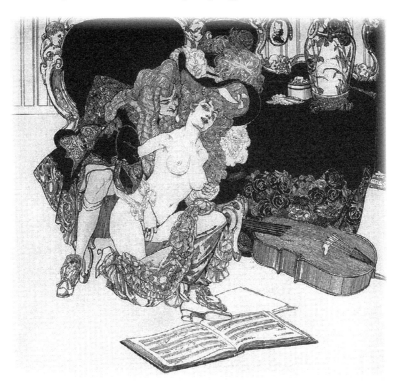

FRANZ VON BAYROS, *late 1800's*

If you stay with it, you'll attain mastery, a state where you no longer need to think about what you're doing—you'll be in deep connection with your sexual instrument, playing delightful improvisations of pleasure. And, once you've developed proficiency with your solo skills, you'll have the expertise to make magic happen when you play duets with others. In fact, you'll be able to knock all your socks right off (and probably the rest of your clothes as well!)

First, though, you have to begin at the beginning.

No Right Way

Please remember this, always: *there is no one right way to do any of this.* You can't do it wrong and you cannot fail. If you get stuck in a loop worrying if you're doing it right, remind yourself that there's no one correct way—there is only what works, or doesn't work, for you.

> *"Good, this is a chance to experience awkwardness and to discover new kinds of mistakes."*
>
> **MARVIN MINSKY**
> *on learning*

Feel free to be . . . *free!* If I lay out an activity, try it the way I suggest and then, if you're so inclined, change it to suit your own impulses or intuitions. Alternatively, invent something new or explore variations. It's all play . . . so play with it!

Beautiful Mistakes

If one thing is certain about your learning journey, it's this—you'll make mistakes. About that, I have just one thing to say: congratulations! Making mistakes is an important part of learning, so try to accept and even embrace them. Yes, you may feel awkward at first. It's only natural. If you appreciate your flubs and blunders as learning opportunities and don't let them deter you, you'll continue to improve. Don't get discouraged by this normal phase of learning new skills—just keep at it and you'll develop competence and confidence. And then discover new kinds of mistakes!

Accept Yourself

You can take this as a first principle of sorts: if you want to be an erotic virtuoso, you need to feel comfortable in and with your body, whatever its size and shape. You must feel secure and unashamed about who you are physically and sexually, which can be a particularly challenging quest in our culture.

We all have a self-critical voice, and sometimes it's turned up so loud we can't hear anything else. Learning to lower the volume (or even turn it off!) is a lifelong practice—and literally a labor of love. I invite you to notice when what I call "Radio Fuck You" is beaming its signal at you. Learn to turn that station off or, even better, to tune in "Radio I Love You." We all know that solo sex is about self-love, so practice speaking kindly to yourself. Whisper sweet nothings into your own hungry ear. And tell that critical bitch to shut up.

Play With It

Remember the way you spontaneously invented games as a child? Let your erotic learning journey be like that—an innocent exploration, a fun voyage, a creative game. These may be "adult" games you're playing, but there's nothing keeping you from bringing to them the creative spirit of a child (other than yourself, that is …).

Life is many things, one of which is a laboratory where we get to conduct ongoing experiments to find out what makes us happy. This is an amazing gift that we've been given. Be grateful. Enjoy the experiments!

Keep the Enchanted Erosphere in Mind

In order to discover our true potential, it helps to know about the vast realm of what's possible, as well as how to get to this enchanted erotic land. It's a lot easier when we have a clear picture of the garden that awaits us.

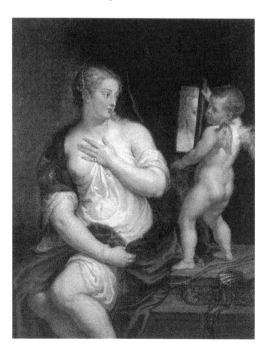

Peter Paul Rubens—*Venus at her Toilet, c. 1600*

Women, you can expand your pathways until you have a multitude of ways to get turned on. You can become *orgasmically proficient*—able to access your orgasm whenever you choose. It then becomes a question of how and how often you'll come, rather than "Will I have one?" You can go on to become *orgasmically abundant*, able to have multiple orgasms with dozens upon dozens of separate peaks, or enter mega-orgasmic states that seem to go on forever. You can train yourself to be able to come from anything, including pleasuring your lover. You can also learn to ejaculate. Men, you can learn to have multiple orgasms without ejaculation (and the satisfaction of knowing you're a master lover!)

All this awaits you in the enchanted Land of Eros. Of course, practice makes perfect, so you probably will have to practice a lot! (Oh, and did I mention the fun you'll have getting there?)

LIBERATE YOUR LANGUAGE

To a significant degree, our language shapes who we are. If our sexual terminology connotes shame and discomfort, then those feelings are part of us.

To free the lover within, you need a language that supports your freedom, a hot sexual vocabulary that's comfortable and clear. Since, as we've already seen, we don't currently have that language, we have to create it. Happily, there's nothing keeping us from doing exactly that.

For starters, you can learn to love, or at least be okay with, the "dirty" words we already know. Personally, I happen to be quite fond of the word "pussy" to describe the female genitalia: after all, they're both furry and fun to pet! The word "cock" works for me, too, although I note with interest that both words refer to domesticated animals. Are we really all that tame? When we free our wild selves, maybe we'll have a wolf and tigress in our pants!

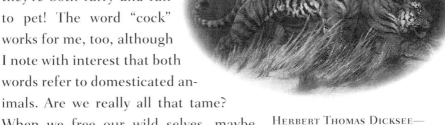

HERBERT THOMAS DICKSEE—
Two Tigers, c. 1900

I'm also quite fond of the word "slut." It's a big-time pejorative for most people, but not me. I use the word to designate anyone, male or female, who loves sex and brings a healthily sex-positive attitude to his or her erotic activities.* "Slut" doesn't mean promiscuous; it means someone sexually free (in a boundary-respecting, appropriate, consensual way, of course!). So, to borrow badly from Shakespeare: what's in a slut? Lots of yummy things, hopefully!

---

* This usage follows the lead of Dossie Easton and Catherine Liszt, authors of the book *The Ethical Slut.*

But I digress. The list of slang words for body parts and sexual activities is vast, so take your prick (er, I mean, pick) and find your favorites. Or, alternatively, find the words that you dislike the least and keep using them until they've lost their charge and simply become the words you use to describe your sexy bits and games.

You can also create your own language or names for your sexual equipment and activities. If your fifi wants to play find the pearl or fetch the frisbee with your sweetie's sweetmeats, then let the games begin! Just remember to clue your partner in to your own personal lexicon. Otherwise, you might wind up with an actual scaloppini canoodling in your swisher when you had something else in mind.

Another option is to borrow language from cultures that revered sex as sacred and structured their vocabulary accordingly. The traditional Indian word for the female genitalia is yoni, which in Sanskrit (the spiritual language of ancient India) means the sacred temple or gate or (my favorite translation) the entrance to the universe. It's a description that makes sense: that's how we got here, after all! The sacred Sanskrit word for male genitalia is the lingam or the vajra. Together, the yoni and the lingam form a blessed altar expressing reverence for the yin-yang nature of reality and our holy power of creation.

Yoni-Lingam Altar, India

To create a sex-positive culture within ourselves, in our relationships and in our world, we need to feel free to talk, to ask, to discuss. I invite you to begin the process by examining your own relationship with words. Is your voice fully liberated? Find the courage to speak your sexual truth, claim your words and start talking. Words are hot! Use them to ask for what you want, turn yourself and your lover on, explore new territory and make your communications sizzle.

Ultimately, it doesn't matter what words you use as long as you're comfortable using them. Words can limit us or set us free. So borrow some, reclaim others or have fun making them up. Do whatever works for you. And remember: every time you speak your sexual truth, you're scoring a point for erotic empowerment!

Making the Most of Your Learning Journey

Here's a summary of the concepts you'll need to derive the most benefit from your learning journey:

- *Know Your Curriculum:* Solo skills are where you start. You'll be using the same skills in partner play, but they're more complex and advanced.

- *Practice Makes Access.* It's natural to make mistakes and feel awkward at first. Don't worry: practice makes proficient.

- *No Right Way.* If the way I suggest doesn't work for you, try another way. There's only one "right way"—the way that works for you.

- *Beautiful Mistakes.* Be okay with making mistakes. You can't learn without them.

- *Accept Yourself.* Be nice to yourself; be positive about yourself. When "Radio Fuck You" starts playing in your head, lower the volume or change the channel.

- *Play With It.* Bring the playful spirit of the child to your learning activities. It really *is* a game . . . especially if you treat it that way!

- *Keep the Enchanted Erosphere in Mind.* Learning can feel like a slog sometimes. When this happens, remember the amazing sex life that awaits you.

- *Liberate Your Language.* Don't let yourself be hamstrung by the limiting language of our culture. Every time you speak about sex in a way that's positive and celebratory, you're claiming your erotic freedom.

Shame-Free Sex: Freeing Your Mind

We all have inhibitions and assumptions that block us from fulfilling our potential. In the sexual realm, these include negative messages we've absorbed from family, friends, media, sex partners and others, as well as the beliefs and defenses we've created in response to our life experiences.

"Emancipate yourself from mental slavery; none but ourselves can free our minds."

BOB MARLEY

To achieve erotic mastery, we need to get rid of these negative messages or, at a minimum, reduce their impact to below the "really screw you up" level. This requires us to haul these old tapes into the light of awareness. Becoming self-aware about our blocks and inhibitions is the first step to becoming truly adept at sex.

You'll need to be patient. We've had years of internalized voices telling us what to do and, perhaps more importantly, what not to do in an endless stream of negativity. You *can* reprogram your brain, but it won't happen overnight. Clearing out baggage takes time, patience and repetition.

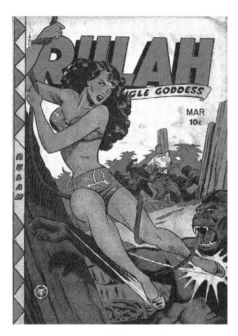

Fox Comics, probably MARK BAKER—
Rulah, Jungle Goddess

COURAGE

To replace these negative messages, you'll need to stand up to the critical voices in your head. Doing this requires self-assertion and, even more fundamentally, courage. I'm not suggesting you have to be fearless. Courage means going ahead and doing it even if you are afraid.

Love yourself well by proceeding gradually. Confronting our negative patterning about sex isn't easy, and courage doesn't require you to jump off the deep end. Even if you sail slowly against the wind of your critical internalized voices, you'll be acting courageously. And remember: once you get in the habit of "doing it anyway," being courageous will only get easier. Courage is like a muscle: the more we use it, the stronger it gets.

"Do one thing every day that scares you."

ELEANOR ROOSEVELT

SAYING YES! GRANTING WILD PERMISSION

Permission is the authorization to allow something. We're taught to look outside ourselves for permission from authorities, parental units, religious institutions and countless other sources of restraint. Complying with external rules is definitely something we need to do, considering that there are these things called laws along with the unqualified need to respect others' boundaries. Unfortunately, alongside these external and important requirements, we also often have unnecessary internalized "shoulds" and "oughts" that block our way.

When it comes to our sexual fulfillment, we must be our own personal authority (while still carefully honoring others' boundaries). When you hear that internalized "No," I encourage you to counter it with a resounding "Yes!" Push back against ingrained negativity. Give yourself permission to be your own boss in deciding what you'll let yourself try or enjoy.

If you notice yourself retreating from your pleasure or blocking your arousal, that's exactly the moment to go for it. Don't brake for that voice in your head! Instead, claim your erotic birthright. Ultimately, you are the only one who can give you permission to be free.

Keep Playing Those Mind Tools Forever

While it's convenient for instructional purposes to treat the mind as its own discrete realm, this isn't actually the case. Science has finally confirmed what ancient wisdom traditions have known for millennia: you can't separate your mind from your body. The idea that our mind is comprised solely of our physical brain and therefore literally

"My brain? It's my second favorite organ."

WOODY ALLEN

"all in your head" is now known to be untrue. In fact, even if we were to expand our definition of "mind" to include all of our neuronal tissue, it still wouldn't be contained inside our cranium because we have an entire nervous system surrounding our gastrointestinal tract, and another tied into our heart.

You may be familiar with the line about our most powerful sex organ being the one between our ears. There's truth in this, but given what we now know about the physiology of mind, it's not quite accurate. It's better put this way: our best sexual asset is a well-hung mind.

Before continuing, I should note that it's not just the mind and body that are connected. All four basic skills—mind and heart, which we discuss in this chapter, and body and spirit, which we explore in Chapter Ten—are interwoven in a single integral unit. I call this framework Wholistic Sexuality for a reason . . .

If you don't, um, mind, we'll begin with the brain. Learning to make the most of this scrumptious erogenous zone is an essential part of your toolkit and a key to expanding your sexuality. There are four mind tools in all: 1) attention and awareness, 2) intention, 3) entrancement and 4) imagination. Let's consider each in turn.

The Mind Tools

AWARENESS AND ATTENTION. We get the most out of our sexual experiences by bringing the full force of our attention to bear on what is happening. Focusing your awareness where you choose is a learned skill—and an ongoing practice.

INTENTION. By consciously setting a clear purpose, you can focus your energy and accelerate the learning process.

ENTRANCEMENT. Sexual arousal is an altered state. You can use your body tools (breath, sound and motion) to maintain and enhance this experience.

IMAGINATION. Imagination is a free zone. Use it to open yourself sexually—and learn about yourself as well!

AWARENESS AND ATTENTION

We are unimaginably complex creatures, living in a world rich with internal and external stimuli. Much of what goes on around and inside us is not accessible to our awareness. You can't feel your liver cleansing your blood, even if you try. Even if we limit ourselves to what we *could* theoretically perceive, we'd still be subjected to an utterly overwhelming amount of information and sensation. This is why we have internal filters that keep most of that deluge below our awareness. If we actually experienced everything that was happening to us, we'd drown beneath the flood.

Your awareness is like a bright flickering screen in a huge shadowy factory with vast mysterious machinery humming away in a thousand dark places. What shows up on the screen is only a tiny fraction of what's actually happening. Everything else stays below, in the black unconscious, the shadowy subconscious and the inaccessible operations of our autonomic systems.

Often, what appears on the screen feels random and outside our control. This is how things seem when we turn over the projector to our "automatic self." When this happens, we're not exercising choice; we simply let it roll.

All else being equal, it's always better to consciously choose what's playing on your internal movie screen. In no small measure, this is because our projectors tend to spend a disproportionate amount of time dredging stuff up from less useful chapters of our past. All too often, ancient self-defeating stories, scratchy old "should" and "ought" recordings and endless babbling about our faults, flaws and inadequacies play in endless re-runs.

We don't have to be totally passive, of course. To some extent, we can control what appears on the screen. We do so—and now we come to the first mind skill—by exercising *awareness* and corralling our *attention*.

If you meditate, you're familiar with this concept. In a nutshell, meditation is about getting better at paying attention. Our mind is like a monkey that spends its time jumping about without focus or discipline. When we meditate, we practice consciously paying attention to what our monkey-mind is doing. It's the consummate meta-activity: we observe ourselves having thoughts, feelings, fantasies and so on. We witness without judgment our mind's wanderings. By doing this diligently, over time we learn to train that mischievous, distractible monkey to do what we want it to do rather than . . . *whatever*.

What does all this have to do with sex? At first blush (not that I blush very much), not much. When we think of meditation, we typically picture someone sitting very still and doing very little. Maybe they're wearing white and sitting on an organic meditation cushion. When we think of sex, the images are usually a tiny bit different . . . as in, likely to involve naked intersecting bodies, lots of grunting and groaning, and the emission of bodily fluids. Doesn't seem spiritual, right? Don't let this fool you. Sex can be a profoundly spiritual activity if we choose to make it so. The fact is, it's a great place to practice meditation-style awareness. It's a great place, in other words, to train our monkey, even if—*especially* if!—he or she is fucking like an, um, animal and howling at the moon.

BAD MOVIES

I strongly encourage you to begin playing with your mind by bringing attention to your mental activities when you're having solo sex. When you do, it's likely that the first thing you'll notice is your mind serving up negative messages. Maybe it's about what's wrong with your body, or perhaps a specific sexual challenge, or something your partner does in bed that you find really annoying. Or maybe it's the argument you had with your mother last week . . . or all of the above!

What you don't want during sex is a screen cluttered up with detrimental messages, chatter about whether you should be behaving this way, or thoughts that block you from moving into the entrancement of arousal. Fears, anxieties and inhibitions can fill that precious screen of awareness with their critical judgments.

GREAT MOVIES

Practicing attention isn't only about showing negative messages the door. It also has a positive aspect—it's about attending to the hot stuff that's going on. Great sex can only happen when you're fully there. Erotic pleasure is one of life's great gifts, but you have to be present to get the present.

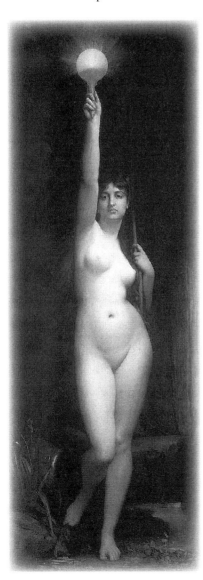

Ideally, not only do you want to be present, but you want to bring all the luscious sensations up onto your brain screen in Technicolor. You want to be exquisitely aware of every little nuance and moment of the pleasure—feeling the flirty hand on your thigh . . . *and* the hot breath against your neck . . . *and* the feel of sweet flesh under your fingers . . . *and* that wonderful musky smell . . . *and* the sunlight pouring through the window. As part of your erotic learning journey, you want, in other words, to cultivate *expanded focus*: you want to experience as much sensation as possible.

To do this, start (as always) with self-awareness. Notice if you're being present or if you've wandered off. When you do drift away (and you will—that's how our monkey minds operate), notice as soon as possible that you're roaming, then lovingly and gently bring yourself back home.

In the next chapter, we'll explore ways to use our body tools to support this practice.

JULES-JOSEPH LEFEBVRE—*Truth*

INTENTION

Whenever we do something, there is always an intention behind it, though usually it's semiconscious, vague and unarticulated. Explicit intentions are quite different. They help us focus our energy and facilitate mani-

Be faithful to that which exists within yourself."

ANDRE GIDE

festation. Setting a conscious intention is an act of choice—you select what you wish to focus on and put it up on your screen in big beautiful letters as a touchstone to keep you on track. Clear intentions focus your unruly mind on where you want it to go. They put a movie title on your screen, acting as a theme to direct the story line.

Play and Practice
Make a List and Check It Twice

Make a list of all the intentions you might want to have in the areas of sexuality and self-love. Here are some of the intentions you may want to use when you play with yourself:

- To relax
- To practice skills
- To have fun
- To see how far you can take yourself out
- To play out particular fantasies.

How many other intentions can you come up with? Keep adding to your list as you come up with new ideas. It's a great way to organize your learning process.

I invite you to bring conscious intention to your sexual self-love sessions. Maybe it's late at night and you just want to have a quickie with yourself to release tension and drift off to sleep in a pleasant post-orgasmic haze. That's a perfectly

"Writing is like making love. Don't worry about the orgasm, just concentrate on the process."

ISABEL ALLENDE

lovely intention and a great way to take care of yourself. However, it's a very different motivation from planning a date with yourself where your intention is to explore your arousal and find out how wild you can get. Neither intention is better than the other. They will, however, produce dramatically different experiences. In your learning journey, use your conscious, focused intention to take you exactly where you want to go.

ENTRANCEMENT

As we saw in Chapter One, arousal is an altered state of consciousness. You come to this place by climbing the ladder of arousal and when you come to your senses—quite literally, in this case—you find yourself . . . not in Kansas anymore. You pass

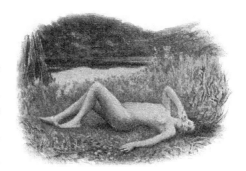

ANONYMOUS—*Daphnis and Chloe, c.1890*

through the *entrance* into a state of *entrancement*, and once you get there, you'll want the experience to be as deep and lasting as possible.

You'll want to—and, despite what it sounds like, this is not the hook of a hip-hop song—"enhance your trance."

This is another place where your basic body toolkit of breath, sound and muscle movement can make a huge difference to enhance and extend your altered state. I'll be discussing this in much greater detail in the next chapter.

IMAGINATION

Your imagination offers many ways to explore and expand your sexuality. In large measure, this is because your brain is, to put it bluntly, gullible. It tends to believe whatever we tell it, even if it's not so. Guys, if you have a wet dream, your brain believes you're actually having sex with those three hotties and—okay, the rest will stay our secret. Women, if you imagine a sexy someone lasciviously licking your slick bits, your body will respond as if it were real because your silly old brain assumes it's so.

Studies have shown that athletes who mentally rehearse perform better than those who don't. It's also been proven that imagining yourself exercising actually improves strength and muscle tone.* What we can glean from this is that you can put your imagination to work (or, rather, to play) for you in the sexual realm. You can use it to:

- Block out distractions, heighten concentration and enhance your erotic trance

- Train your brain, hone your responses and help you quickly learn new pathways to orgasm and arousal

- Re-program negative mind-tapes.

We all have lots of inner material to work with. You can visualize body processes such as the puffing and ripening of your yoni and its erectile circuits (or—let's be gender-neutral here—other swelling processes). You can also work with ideas, images and stories.

The power of fantasy can't be overstated. The stories you use to turn yourself on can be things you've actually experienced, things you'd like to experience or things you'd never dream of actually trying in real life. That's one of the great things about fantasy: it doesn't come with a contract saying you have to do it.

---

* Unfortunately, you'll get much more buff if you actually exercise.

Your Magic Mind Movie

If you're like most of us, you probably spend a lot of time imagining various possible futures as well as re-visioning your past. You can use this propensity to heal, learn and explore. Because the brain is so gullible, it will believe the stories you tell it.

One particularly powerful way to do this is with *guided imagery* or *visualization*. Basically, you tell yourself a story and experience it with your inner eye or other senses. For some, imaginary life is a very visual experience while others imagine sensations, tastes, textures, sounds, words or energy. Use whatever works best for you—and, ideally, employ as many modalities as possible to spin the richest possible inner tales. Here are some suggested mind-movie scripts:

- Use your inner eye to see and amplify what's happening in your body. This is especially wonderful to do with your genitals!

- Play with yourself while wearing a blindfold. Turn your vision inside to see what's happening and focus on feeling all of your exquisite sensations.

- Weave a mental story where you explore new territory.

- Rehearse a potentially anxious situation.

- Think of a new way that you'd like to learn to get off and practice it.

I strongly encourage you to adopt a *no mind-crime* policy. Give your fantasies permission to travel wherever they want to go. Your social behavior requires proper restraints, but your fantasy life doesn't. (In your private storytelling, you may want to include restraints of a different kind, though!)

"Forget safety. Live where you fear to live. Destroy your reputation. Be notorious. I have tried prudent planning long enough. From now on, I'll be mad."

RUMI

We all have notions of what is and isn't appropriate. When you go into sexual fantasy, please park those notions at the door. You might even want to imagine a sign at the entrance to your personal screening-room: "Cultural, religious and politically correct taboos not welcome here."

Your Fantasy Land can be a totally free zone . . . but only if you give it permission. I invite you to exercise your courage muscle by

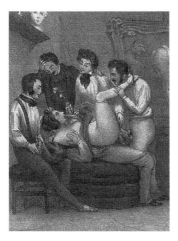

ANONYMOUS—*Postcard, c.1850*

stretching past old limitations and following your desires into forbidden realms. Not only may it turn out to be fabulous fun (busting through boundaries has its own special thrill), but you may well discover new and fascinating things about yourself.

The fact is, the imagination offers enormous learning as well as erotic opportunities. When you go out—*way, way out*—you're giving a hot and invaluable gift to yourself.

Play and Practice
Using Your Imagination

As always, you'll want to start with self-awareness. Tune in and notice where you're blocked and what inhibitions keep you from expressing your wild and free authentic self. For this exercise, choose one specific area that you want to change. For most of us, there's an endless list to choose from—possibilities include body image issues, the use of certain types of words, prohibitions about playing with toys, or exploring forbidden imaginary realms.

Once you've made your choice, turn your focus inward with your breath and use your intention to get centered. Now imagine a scenario in which you do the taboo action. See yourself freely doing it . . . and *loving* it. Imagine your most integrated, bold and wild self acting without shame or guilt. Visualize a real or imaginary partner finding what you're doing a complete turn-on. Breathe in the images and feelings that arise. If inhibitions intrude, acknowledge them and let them go. Breathe them out of your body and then return to the fantasy. Keep claiming your inner freedom.

Heart Skills—Integrating Self-Love and Sex

Many people don't realize that knowing how to love is a set of learnable skills. Some of us were fortunate enough to be raised in an environment where we were seen, honored and respected—and thus learned how to be compassionate, forgiving, generous and open-hearted. Most of us weren't so lucky, though. We learned some good love skills from

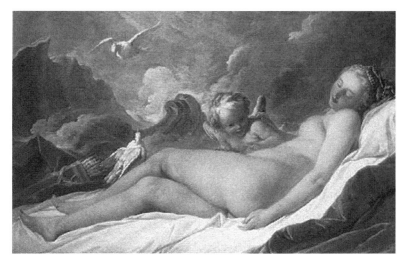

François Boucher—*Le Sommeil de Venus, c. 1750*

our elders while others went begging. More unfortunately still, many of us learned how to be quite actively unloving as we were unconsciously taught to harbor negative attitudes toward ourselves and others.

We all long to love and be loved, but we lack the training to do these things as well as we might— and some of us lack the training to do it even passably. We could all use some remedial love training.

> *"We are shaped and fashioned by what we love."*
>
> GOETHE

Heart skills are what help us love well. As usual, the best place to start is with yourself. Some people confuse self-love with narcissism and view it as selfish or indulgent. It's neither. You can't have a healthy relationship with anyone unless you love yourself.

Unfortunately, many of us are not particularly skilled at loving ourselves well. This hardly comes as a surprise, given that we have a cultural epidemic of low self-esteem. Even among those of us who have a mostly healthy ego, there's usually a piece of us that feels unworthy and has been disowned.

> *"The greatest happiness of life is the conviction that we are loved, loved for ourselves, or rather loved in spite of ourselves."*
>
> VICTOR HUGO

We often compensate for these negative feelings by looking to others for the care, respect and appreciation we crave. If we don't love ourselves, that's a losing proposition. We can't take in love if we don't feel worthy of it.

The Heart Tools

- WITNESSING
- OPEN-HEARTEDNESS
- RESPECT
- COMPASSION AND FORGIVENESS
- GIVING AND RECEIVING
- LOVING INTENTION
- LOVING ACTION

Whole Lotta Loving Going On

Here's a more in-depth yet brief look at the tools and skills of the heart.

WITNESSING

When you see purely, without attaching a narrative or bias, you are witnessing. In order to love clearly and cleanly, we must see ourselves and others as we really are, in all our strength and weakness, beauty and challenges, as whole and complex beings—with acceptance and without judgment.

OPEN-HEARTEDNESS

It seems our egos need to find fault with others. It's our way of reassuring ourselves that we're okay—if they're down, that must mean we're up! Of course, the one we often find the most fault with is actually ourselves (although we conveniently tend to project that onto others). When we practice generosity and open-heartedness, instead of finding fault, we accept and understand.

R-E-S-P-E-C-T

When we dishonor or disrespect others, we're putting them below us—and, alternatively, if we put them above us, it's ourselves we're treating disrespectfully. Respect always begins with ourselves: we begin by treating ourselves with reverence and valuing our own needs. To love well, we then follow the good old golden rule and offer the same honor and respect to others.

Compassion and Forgiveness

When we're on the receiving end of aggravating or disappointing behavior, we basically have two choices. We can get angry and judgmental, or we can be compassionate and forgive. Guess which is the heart skill! And who do we often have the hardest time forgiving? That's right—ourselves. We may find it hard to forgive—we only get good at it when we make compassion an ongoing practice.

Giving and Receiving

People tend to think that loving is all about giving, but it's just as much about receiving. This is because, when we allow ourselves to receive, we're giving to ourselves. (Come to think of it, from this perspective, it actually is all about giving!)

Loving Intention

In any given transaction, we can choose to intend to love. We may not be able to actually pull it off, but our loving intention can be a compass, helping us navigate past the many temptations that can cause us to fall out of loving kindness.

Loving Action

Intention is a great beginning, but it's not enough. You need to practice loving actions, too. Show the love in your conduct toward yourself and others. Take action to take care of yourself. Behave in ways that nurture you!

Love Lists

Love starts at home, with you. One way to start cultivating self-love is by compiling a running list of all the things about you that are wonderful, lovable and positive. Put the list on your altar or refrigerator and refer to it when you're feeling down about yourself. What's to love? A lot!

Here's another useful list: set down all the things you can do to nurture yourself, or to receive support and care from others. Keep adding to the list, and put it where you (and others) can see it.

Don't stop here. Don't just list. *Do.*

We all have the physical equipment for casual sexual encounters, and many of us have the emotional capacity, too. While quickies like this can be wonderfully naughty and delightful, for sex to reach its transcendent potential, we have to show up—and open up—in our entirety. The moral of this story is that the best sex happens when you're making love, even if it's "only" to yourself.

> *"You yourself, as much as anybody in the entire universe, deserve your love and affection."*
>
> **BUDDHA**

Play and Practice
The Perfect Lover Inventory

Take a few moments to imagine your perfect lover. Make a list of this person's qualities and attributes. What does this tell you about what you value most? What do you most desire in a partner?

Once you've finished, ask yourself how similar you are to the person you've just described. Congratulate yourself for the qualities you currently possess. As for the areas where you fall short of the ideal, take a moment and be thankful for what you've just learned. You've just identified some important growth opportunities.

End by appreciating the many qualities you share with your ideal lover.

Loving yourself well takes courage, practice and perseverance. You can choose to be a great self-lover by accessing every bit of pleasure that you're capable of—it's a radical act.

Let's continue our journey by exploring the other tools in your toolkit that will help you cultivate erotic mastery.

CHAPTER TEN

Coming to Your Senses

"The mind's first step to self-awareness
must be through the body."

GEORGE SHEEHAN

A Wholistic Toolkit

IN CHAPTER NINE, WE EXAMINED MIND TOOLS in depth, and heart skills more briefly. Now, we turn our attention to the other two major skill sets—physical and spiritual.

Collectively, these four toolkits are deeply wholistic; along with energy, which I discuss in Chapter Eleven, they provide an integral map that supports both self-awareness and personal learning.

Your three main body tools are breath, sound and movement. Ideally, with practice, you'll get to the point where they all automatically work together during your erotic activities. This "triple play" can become a new baseline for you in revving up your erotic energy; it's like trading in a compact for a sports car.

You can expand your abilities further by adding the other three body tools—vision, touch, and smell/taste. But the three most essential ones are breath, sound and movement.

Begin With Breath

Breath is basic. You don't have to remember any complicated, esoteric formulas or worry if you're doing it wrong, and you certainly won't forget to do it. Breath happens.

Our respiratory system is unique: it's the only place in your body that's innervated by both the voluntary and the involuntary parts of your nervous system. What this means, in a nutshell, is that breath is both autonomic—we breathe without thinking—and also subject to our conscious control—we can ramp it up, hold it and play with it in a multitude of ways.

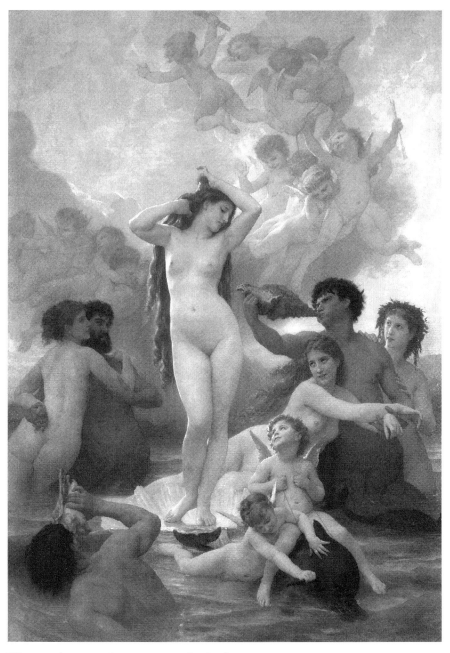

WILLIAM ADOLPHE BOUGUEREAU—*Birth of Venus, c.1870*

When you're not paying attention to your breath, your respiratory pattern will tamely follow your state of being. For example, when you get turned on, you breathe faster as your arousal pulls your breath along behind it. If you want to use your breath consciously, you can do so by flipping the sequence and having your breath pull your arousal along. Deployed this way, breath can propel you to ecstasy.

The Body Tools

The three most foundational skills in your body toolkit are breath, sound and movement:

- BREATH is a bridge you use to shift your energy and state of consciousness. It connects your conscious and unconscious selves and transports you to altered states of arousal.

- SOUND is your internal amplifier of sensation. You can use sound to move sexual energy to specific parts of your body, or to expand and fill your whole body.

- MOVEMENT increases circulation, stimulates your nerves and engages the more animal parts of your brain. It stirs the subtle flow of our life force. The most fundamental erotic movements involve our internal and external pelvic muscles.

The other three body skills are vision, touch and taste/smell:

- VISION in the solo context is mostly about *inner vision*. Use it to hone in on your inner experience and to do visualizations that empower you and increase your erotic abilities.

- There are four types of TOUCH: nurturing, therapeutic, sensual and erotic.

- SMELL is our prime signal for mating. It opens up the pathways to sensual experience. TASTE and smell are closely related. We can only differentiate among five types of taste—bitter, salty, sweet, sour and spicy.

ENHANCE IT TILL YOU DANCE IT

When you lead your arousal with your breathing, do so gently. Don't fake it by using giant, exaggerated breath patterns. "Fake it till you make it" won't work here. It just leaves you feeling inauthentic and dysfunctional, and if you have a partner, it will create a false baseline for communication with that person. Instead, use your toolkit to enhance and amplify your state. Simply nudge your arousal along by enhancing whatever breathing pattern is happening naturally. Breathe a little deeper or pick up the speed a bit. Don't try to force your breath way out ahead of your arousal—just send it a pace or two out in front. Wait till your energy catches up with your breath, then repeat. Keep on doing this to climb the arousal ladder. Over time, you can learn to take this all the way to orgasm.

Generally, you'll want to breathe faster to increase tension and accelerate your arousal. However, since arousal is a delicate dance between tension and relaxation, occasionally you'll want to slow and deepen your breathing instead. Play with both; there is no right way.

You can use your mouth or nose for the inhale or the exhale, making four possible patterns in all. Here, too, there is no correct method. The ancient erotic traditions actually give conflicting guidance about this! Do what works best for you, bearing in mind that different pathways will tend to generate different states. In general, start with what's most comfortable, then try it another way and notice the difference. Breathing through your mouth tends to be a more primal pathway, so I especially encourage you to explore breath play with a relaxed jaw, an open throat and a softly open mouth.

"The sexual embrace can only be compared with music and with prayer."

MARCUS AURELIUS
(Roman emperor, AD 121–180)

Your mouth and throat are one end of a channel—the other end is your pelvic floor and genitalia. This connection means that when your mouth and throat are loose and open, your pelvic area is also able to relax and open, allowing your erotic energy to flow freely. You might want to imagine yourself as having a tube or pipe that runs from your mouth to your pelvic region. You won't be the first person to do this: all the energy systems handed down to us by primal peoples include this sort of channel.

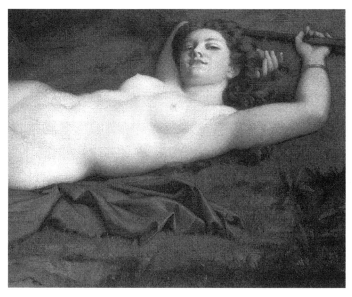

PIERRE HONORE HUGREL—*Bacchante—detail, c.1870*

As you breathe, notice what's happening with your face, your mouth and throat as well as your pelvic area. Keep both territories loose and relaxed.

Play and Practice
Basic Breath Practices

Here are some basic breath practices to get you started on the path to more pleasure:

- *Breath Awareness Practice.* The next few times you're taking matters into your own hands, be aware of how you breathe while in the various stages of your journey. That's all you need to do: simply pay attention and notice what happens when.

- *Breath Augmentation.* If you want a simple way to increase and deepen your arousal, and also extend and expand your orgasms, simply enhance whatever your breath is already doing by itself. A little will go a long way here. Breathe a little faster, draw it in a little deeper, let it out a bit longer, or open your chest and belly more. Play with ways to enhance your natural patterns. Notice what happens.

- *Mouthing Off.* Breathe in and out through your mouth. Try using loosely pursed lips for the inhale and a relaxed loosely open mouth for the exhale. Practice awareness of your breath as you do this. Try it at different levels of your arousal journey and notice your response.

- *Accelerating Breath.* To raise your energy and build arousal, start with slow deep breaths. Breathe all the way down into your belly. Gradually deepen the breath and increase the pace while continuing to pull the breath into your belly. Keep getting faster until you're panting deeply and rapidly. Notice how you feel as you breathe faster. Slow down when you need to and let your breath calm down. Practice cycles of firing up your breath and cooling it down.

- *Pant and Big Draw.* To ramp up your energy, do a deep, fast, panting breath using your belly muscles for thirty seconds. Imagine fire or heat glowing in your center. Next take two or three deep, long, slow breaths. Imagine you're drawing the energy up on the inhale and moving it down on the exhale, sending it through your whole body. Repeat the pattern of rapid breathing followed by deep draws. Do several cycles. Notice how you feel.

Was it good for you? Or interesting? Great! Now, just breathe . . .

Aural Sex

Your next foundational instrument is your ability to make sexy sounds. I'm not talking about sexy *words* ("cock," "pussy") here; I'm talking about sexy *sounds* ("mmm," "aah"). Words are great for many things, including erotic communication, boundary check-ins and more—but they activate the thinking part of your brain. This is why there's such a big difference between "dirty talk" and lusty sounds. All conceptual

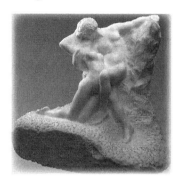

AUGUSTE RODIN—*Eternal Spring*

language, including the stuff you can't say on radio or TV, uses our higher brain centers. Sound emerges from a much more primal place. Being verbally lewd can be spectacularly sexy, but it's gutter sexy, not brain-basement sexy.

Sound also helps you turn off the yammering talk radio station in your mind. You know the voice: it's the one that's always planning, pondering and judging, and virtually impossible to shut up. You need to turn it off, though, if you're going to get turned on. Sound does this by taking you down to where words can't go.

Sound is the Swiss army knife of your tool box. It can do a lot of different things:

- LIGHT UP YOUR BRAIN MAP. When you make sound, it notifies your brain to pay close attention to the really good stuff that's happening right now ... *omigod, right there!* It's your internal attention focus device, amplifying your perception of sensation.

- SHUT YOUR RADIO! As noted above, sound overwrites our endless inner monologue and sends us down a bioelectric elevator to the basement where the ancient machinery responsible for arousal resides. *"Does my ass look fat?" "Is he bored?" "I really need to dust the ceiling!"* Thoughts like these get drowned out by our soundtrack of "ohh" and "aah."

- ATTUNING IN. Sound also creates harmonic resonances with your body and your partner's at every level from the cellular up. It attunes your energy fields and bodily rhythms and helps you connect with yourself and others.

- THE TIMBRE OF TURN-ON. Sexy sound is a huge turn-on for yourself and anyone you're playing with. The more sound you express, the more your pleasure is evident to everyone involved (and sometimes to your neighbors!). Sound creates a positive internal feedback loop—hot makes hotter, you might say—and it's also a great way to turn your partner on while letting him or her know what's working (or not) for you. When you narrate your arousal with sound, you're plugging your partner into your erotic story line.

- SOUNDING UP THE AROUSAL STAIRWAY. Sound can move up or down, or in or out, and as it does, it carries your energy with it. You can use sound to move sexual energy to specific parts of your body or to fill your entire body.

I'm With Stupid

The fact that we're in an altered (and primal) state when aroused explains why conversations about intentions, boundaries, safety and so on need to occur when we're not turned on. It's been said that men only think with their dick. There's some truth in this—and it's also

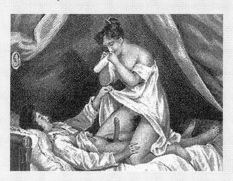

NICOLAS TASSAERT—*The Cautious Lover*

true that women sometimes think with their pussies. How many women have blurted out, "Never mind about a condom!" and risked pregnancy (and disease) because they were down in the brain-basement when they said it and thinking about one thing only—penetration?

The familiar, morning-after, "I can't believe I was so stupid" experience is as common as it is because *sex makes you stupid*. This isn't personal and it's not gender-related, either. It's what has to happen in order for you to have hot sex. The planning and judging center has to go offline and the executive office lights must get turned off for your erotic equipment to get turned on.

High arousal is no time for adult decisions. Discuss, plan and make agreements when your executive higher-level brain is functioning. Prevent morning-after-itis!

SHUSH! SOMEONE MAY HEAR YOU!

We have tremendous sexual sound inhibition in our culture.

Most of us began our sexual journey needing to hide what we were doing, and feeling awkward and inhibited about releasing our pleasure soundtrack. Maybe you didn't want your parents to know what subject you were really studying in your bedroom with your friend, or you didn't want the kids in the front of the car to know what you were up to in the back seat. After that, perhaps you were quiet because you didn't want your roommate to hear. Then there were your kids and the neighbors, then the grandchildren, and then, guess what, you're dead and you spent your whole life silencing your sexual sound track . . . *for what?*

As part of your journey into erotic mastery, I invite you to break free from our pervasive cultural embarrassment about the sounds of sex. I guarantee you, you sound beautiful when you're moaning with pleasure. Anyone who hears the music of your arousal is getting as much of a gift as if you were singing a beautiful song.

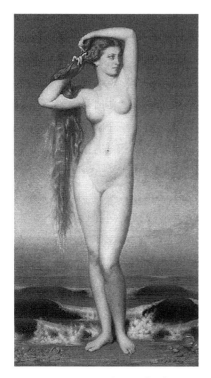

AMAURY DUVAL—*The Birth of Venus*

GO SOUND OFF!

When you first begin to use your sounds, it may feel artificial or awkward. Don't let that stop you! You don't have to turn the volume up to full blast (that can come, so to speak, later), but please do let your sound out, even if only a little, then slowly ramp it up over time. Expressing your freedom this way feels really great—and it's also a wonderful way to exercise your courage muscle.

At first, you may need to force yourself to make sounds. That's okay. Start with little moans, small sighs and soft purrs. Try out different sounds; find out what feels natural. It will get easier as well as hotter over time. Soon, you'll find that there's a whole range of sounds within you and you don't need to think about it anymore. It will just come out when you let it. Release the soundtrack of your pleasure and you'll soar on the sexy sounds!

Sounding, Sighing and Singing

Sound amplifies sensation and expands your experience. It also narrates and communicates your pleasure. To explore your sound possibilities, try the following:

- Make as many different sounds as you can. Moan, sigh, whimper, croon … try to come up with sounds there aren't words for!

- Make open-mouthed sounds with a loose throat. (Notice what happens in your pelvic area when your mouth and throat are tight.) Make a point of staying loose and open.

- Utter different vowels and repeat them, making it sound sexier each time.

- Use sound to express awe, love and agreement. How much can you say without words?

- Make a sound quietly, then repeat it, gradually getting louder each time.

- Experiment with the length of the sound. Is longer better? There's no right answer. Discover what's right for you.

- Put on music and make sounds along with it. (I'm a big fan of ecstatic Sufi music for this!)

- Make animal noises.

- Play with varying the pitch. Highly recommended: sounds that fall, getting deeper and more guttural. This kind of sound moves sexual energy down your body into your crotch.

Moving into Ecstasy

Our next body tool is movement. Muscle activity increases circulation, stimulates your nerves and engages the more animal parts of your brain. It circulates erotic energy, intensifying and raising it. Our gross body movement stirs the subtle flow of our life force.

Our most essential erotic movements involve our internal pelvic muscles. Other foundational motions include pelvic rocking, spinal undulation, vibration and shaking movements. Let's start with our internal pelvic pump.

PELVIC POWER

As noted in Chapter Seven, the base of our body is composed of the pelvic floor muscles. These muscles fill the bottom of our bony pelvis and keep our insides from falling out. They include all of the muscles that control peeing. pooping and reproducing—they hold, squeeze, pull up and in, open, release and push.

The pelvic floor muscles are the basic pump and powerhouse of your sexual gateway. They act like a sort of sexual trampoline, bouncing and rebounding your sexual energy. They can send the current of erotic energy wherever you want it to go.

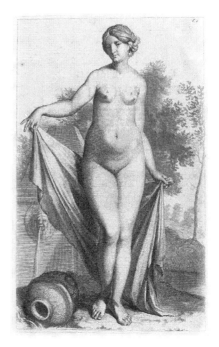

GOVARD BIDLOO, 1690

You can use your inner pelvic muscles to plump up your plumbing. When you pulse your internal pump, you push blood into the erectile tissue, swelling your hard-on or hard-around. Basically, every time you clench and release your pelvic floor muscles, you're playing with yourself without using your hands. This is a very useful skill, since your hands are often busy playing with other things.

Play and Practice
The Elevator

In addition to being able to tighten and release, your pelvic floor muscles can push. When you poop or give birth, you're using this ability. You can practice opening your bottom and pushing, which can come in handy not just for bodily functions, but also for propelling your orgasmic energy.

An exercise called "The Elevator" is a good way to learn how to control your pelvic floor muscles as well as how to push them down and open your bottom up.

Imagine that your pelvic floor is an elevator in a building with three stories and a basement. Start at the first floor, which is neutral and relaxed. Partially draw the floor muscles up and together, as if you were taking the elevator to the second floor. Hold for a moment. Draw the muscles completely tight, as far up as possible. That's the third floor. Again, hold for a moment. Now let the elevator back down to the partially contracted state (the second floor). Relax back down to the neutral state of the first floor, then push down and out with your muscles: your "elevator" is now descending to the basement. Push with your belly muscles and diaphragm as if you're having a big poop. Accompany your visit to the basement with a deep, grunting exhalation.

Repeat.

These muscles are a key to expanding your sexual response. Plus, being able to use them well will make your partners, who may have parts of themselves inside you, very happy.

"And the day came when the risk it took to remain tight inside the bud was more painful than the risk it took to blossom."

ANAIS NIN

Play and Practice
The Jade Egg

Women, imagine having a smooth, oval, warm egg-shaped stone nestled in the lips of your yoni. Use your muscles to move the imaginary egg. Imagine that you are sucking the egg up and inside yourself, slowly rolling it up the vaginal canal until it rests at the cervix, then moving it back down and push it out. Make sounds while you do the movements. Repeat as many times as you like, for as long as feels good.

In the Taoist tradition, women use an oval jade stone for these exercises. If you'd like to train your pelvic floor muscles using something more tangible than your imagination, you can buy a jade egg or make your own equivalent, using a pleasing smooth stone or egg-shaped crystal. You can also use a dildo or other toy—and, if you have access to a willing cock, you can also play with pulling it into you, holding and squeezing it, and pushing it out again.

OTHER MOTIONS

Other types of motion can also facilitate arousal.

There is the *pelvic rock*, which is the basic mammalian fucking motion. Rocking and thrusting the hips—okay, *humping*!—pumps cerebral-spinal fluid, activates our animal brain and stimulates multiple nerve pathways. These rhythmic movements will release your orgasmic energy, especially when enhanced by breathing. So loosen up your hips and let them rock and roll!

Your *spine* is another key to easier arousal and heightened orgasmic power. When it's loose, an undulating wave of energy (known in the Indian tradition as *kundalini*) can ripple up and down your body's core.

Full body vibration, including *shaking* and *rhythmic oscillation*, is another pathway for ecstatic energy. These are natural movements, although many of us have had these instinctual responses blocked by cultural conditioning. You can learn to reconnect and open to your natural erotic vibration.

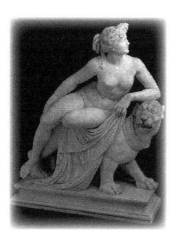

Ancient Greece—Cybele Riding the Lion

Putting Your Big Three
Body Tools Together

Once you've got a handle on the basic motion skills, especially the ones involving the pelvic floor muscles, you can begin to play with coordinating your bottom and your breath. The following exercise has multiple variations.

BREATHING THROUGH YOUR BOTTOM. Start with a basic pelvic pump. This time, though, coordinate the pulsing motion with your breath. Imagine your breath flowing in and out through your bottom as you pump your pelvic floor muscles.

You have two options here: you can tighten on the inhale or the exhale. Notice which pattern is natural for you. While there is no right way (yes—that point again!), the two patterns do tend to have different effects.

- *Connection Pattern.* Tighten with the inhale and release with the exhale. Usually this helps you be present and centered in your body.

- *Pump It Up Pattern.* Open your bottom on the inhale and pull up on the exhale. This pattern tends to fuel arousal. This pattern is especially useful when you want to ramp your medium-level arousal up to high.

Start with whichever is easiest and more natural for you. Then try the reverse pattern to see what that feels like.

ADD SOUND. After you've become adept at synching your breath with your basic pelvic floor movements, try the same exercises and add sound to your exhale. Play with different sounds and discover which ones most help you connect and coordinate your actions.

These are three key tools—breath, movement and sound. Experiment with different ways to use them together!

"This Being of mine, whatever it really is, consists of a little flesh, a little breath, and the part which governs."

MARCUS AURELIUS

Use Your Body-Mind
Skills to Come Home

If you notice you're not being fully present, you can bring your mind back home by using your breath, sound and pelvic floor muscles in combination.

As soon as you realize that your mind has gone a-roving, inhale a big lungful of air while pulling up your pelvic floor muscles. Then exhale, accompanying the out-breath with sound, as you relax your muscles and send the energy down your spine and out your crotch. Repeat this until you are fully back in your body. The simple process of taking five or ten deep, sounding breaths while opening and closing your pelvic floor is an effective training device for your monkey mind.

Then dip into your basic toolkit and pull out your sound. This delivers a message to your brain: "Something good is happening. Pay attention!" Making sound floods your mind with sexy stimulation while drowning out critical voices.

I See! The Power of Visioning

Our next skill set is vision—and since we're focusing on self-skills, I'm referring to our *inner* vision. What happens when you close your eyes and look inside? To some extent, that depends on who you are. Some of us see color, lights or patterns. Others see energy channels, the vortexes of our energy centers, or images of divine beings. Or, you might be one of those people with little ability to see pictures of any sort, but who can feel vibration or sense movement.

> The ear tends to be lazy, craves the familiar, and is shocked by the unexpected: the eye, on the other hand, tends to be impatient, craves the novel and is bored by repetition.
>
> W.H. AUDEN

Visualizations are a great way to use your inner vision. When we do this, we decide what we're going to see and then we instruct our mind to see it. Visualizations are particularly effective when we combine them with the three basic body tools of breath, sound and motion.

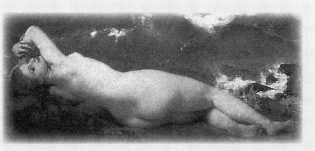

PAUL JACQUES-AIME BAUDRY— *The Wave and the Pearl, mid 1800's*

Play and Practice
A Sampling of Visualizations

WAVE BREATH. Use this practice to relax, get present or deepen your arousal. Do slow, deep breaths. Imagine your exhale beginning in the center of your body and rolling outward in a circular wave, like a ripple from a stone thrown into a pond. Visualize (and feel) your inhale as the circular wave flowing back into your center.

OPENING THE TUBE. Use this practice to connect your mouth, throat and nose with your pelvic area. Breathe through an open mouth, using loosely pursed lips for the inhale and a loose open mouth for the exhale. (Breathing in through your nose is okay, too, although try to keep using your opened mouth for the exhale. You can also try inhaling with both nose and mouth and see which works better for you.)

Imagine a tube or inner channel that runs up the center of your body. On the inhale, imagine your breath flowing in your mouth and all the way down and out your bottom. On the exhale, see and feel your breath flowing into your bottom and out your mouth. Try to experience your whole internal channel as breathing.

As you bring this image into focus, notice how the tube looks and feels. Is it open or constricted? Are some parts open and others tight? Is there color, light, heat or vibration? Is there a sense or image of movement? Try adding sounding breaths and pumping your pelvic floor muscles—can you expand the tube more? Can you create a sense or vision of energy moving? Try some of the following visualizations:

- See particles or colors or light moving up and down the conduit.

- Imagine the channel filled with different colors.

- See something representing earth energy flowing in the bottom and divine energy flowing in and out the top.

Take a few moments to visualize your inner pathway as open and energized. End with a few deep centering breaths.

(continued on next page)

SEEING WHAT'S SO. Before beginning the physical part of the exercise, take some time to review this book's images of female anatomy. Now close your eyes. Center yourself with a few deep, slow breaths. Bring your awareness down into your genitals. Now send your breath down there. Make some soft opening sounds. Gently pulse your pelvic floor muscles and rock your hips. Take a few moments to feel really good about all of your delicious parts.

Now focus on visualizing exactly what you have from the inside. Notice each separate part and send loving sound and breath into each delectable bit of you. Play with your pelvic floor muscles as you focus on the various aspects of your anatomy. Bring your awareness to the outer lips. Imagine them opening like a flower as you breathe and pulse them open. Send sounding breaths into your inner lips as you visualize them opening and blooming. Imagine the entrance to your vagina as a cuff and play with clenching and releasing it. Go deeper inside and imagine your vaginal canal pulsing, opening and closing, pulling in and pushing out. Bring your awareness to your bladder and urethra and then to your uterus, playing with each part in turn. Bring your attention to your anus, pulsing it as you make sounding breaths.

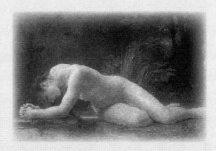

WILLIAM ADOLPHE BOUGUEREAU—
Biblis, mid 1800's

Conclude your experience by taking a few moments to visualize your genitals being held, loved and revered. End with a few deep centering breaths.

The Art of Touch

Touch is one of our first languages of love and a universal form of communication. It's also one of our earliest senses; it was already active when you were swimming in the womb. It's a profoundly primal need: babies will die without the nourishment of skin contact. In large measure due to our cultural anxiety about sex, most of us don't get anywhere near the touch we need. Even if we're getting lots of sex, we can still have a touch deficit.

"The nice thing about masturbation is that you don't have to dress up for it."

TRUMAN CAPOTE

How often do you practice self-touch? Many people hardly touch themselves at all. When you do, is your touch limited to your sex parts? Do you massage yourself? Hold or hug yourself? Do you comfort yourself with touch?

There are four basic types of touch:

- *Nurturing touch* communicates love and acceptance. It's how a doting parent touches their baby.

- *Therapeutic touch* is about healing. It eases pain and stress.

- *Sensual touch* heightens the senses, amplifies our bodily awareness and promotes physical pleasure.

- *Sexual touch* fires us up erotically.

When you touch yourself, please don't limit yourself to your juicy bits and other erogenous zones! I'm certainly not counseling you against spending plenty of time playing with yourself sexually. I'm a sex teacher, after all! But you also need to not give short shrift to the other three types of touch. You can love yourself with all four kinds of touch, and I encourage you to do so.

I urge you to bring the same skill, imagination and intention to your self-pleasuring touch that you would to pleasuring a lover. Touch everything: after all, it's yours! Run your hands through your hair, stroke your belly, rub your neck, tease your nipples. Use your basic body skills of breath, sound and pelvic pump to fully receive what you're giving yourself. How present can you be for yourself?

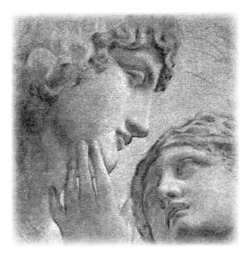

ANONYMOUS—*Eros and Psyche*

Touching Is for Earthlings, Feeling Is for Martians

There's a big difference between *touching* and *feeling*. When you touch something, you experience it more abstractly and less intimately than if you're feeling it. Touch is mediated by all sorts of expectations and assumptions. For instance, if you're touching skin, the experience is mediated by your awareness of what skin is supposed to feel like, and also how you're supposed to touch it in order to touch it "well." There's nothing wrong with this sort of touch, but it lacks a certain specialness. It lacks what Zen practitioners call beginner's mind.

Feeling something is very different. It's like the first time, every time.

You can discover the difference by playing the following game with yourself. First, choose a part of your body and touch it. Don't make a big deal out of it. Caress it, squeeze it . . . make contact with it in the ways you normally would.

Now pretend that you're a Martian and this is your first encounter with an Earthling. You've never encountered skin before; your language doesn't even have a word for it! Now touch this same part of yourself. Explore it with the curiosity and innocence you'd bring to a totally (and literally) alien experience.

When you've finished, take a few moments to register the difference between touching, which is what you did on the first round, and feeling, which is what your Martian *alter ego* did. If you wish, jot down some notes.

There is nothing wrong with touching. We do it all the time, and it's fine. Feeling, however, has a magical sensuous quality that standard-issue touching lacks. When you're practicing touch (and I'm using it in the generic sense here), make a point of folding feeling into your repertoire.

Juicy Pleasures—Taste and Smell

It's a little-known fact that taste is a very simple sense. All it can do is differentiate among sweet, sour, salty, bitter and spicy. All the rest of the complexities of taste are mediated by smell, which bypasses the higher-level and relatively new neocortex and is connected directly to our old brain.

For most mammals, smell is the prime signal for mating. The ancient mating signals of scent and pheromones, the less obvious chemical signals, all enter through our nasal passages. We even have a bit of erectile tissue around our nostrils. When we're turned on, we tune in to smell. Conversely, when we consciously engage our sense of smell, we open to our sensual experience and stimulate the lower arousal part of our brain. Hooray for strawberries and chocolate!

Play and Practice
Yum, Yum, YUM!

You can do this exercise with your eyes open, closed or blindfolded.

Gather a diverse selection of tasty goodies. Begin by leisurely smelling each of them. First, do so without making any sound, then repeat while making sounds of pleasure and appreciation.

Now enhance your breath. Notice the difference when you add these body tools.

Repeat the process, only this time with tasting. Savor the smell and then take a nibble, bringing all of your awareness to your mouth, tongue and teeth. Eat it slowly, consciously experiencing the various flavors and textures.

Repeat the tasting process a second time, this time adding your pleasure soundtrack and enhanced breath. Notice any differences.

Using Everything You've Got

We've now reviewed your six body tools—breath, sound, movement, vision, touch, and smell/taste. I encourage you to practice using them all, and not according to a schedule. Use any of the tools whenever it occurs to you to do it. When you sink into a hot bath, let out moans of

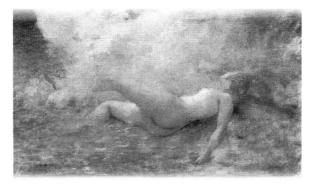

HENRI GERVEX—*Woman Tossed by a Wave, c. 1890*

pleasure. When you go out of your house on a crisp autumn morning, take a moment to do deep breathing. Sigh as you stretch into a yoga posture and give your pelvic floor some sweet squeezes.

In addition, bring your toolkit into your erotic play. Use all your tools, with special attention to your primary body toolkit of breath, sound and movement. The more you practice these skills, the better you'll get at tuning into your experience, accelerating your arousal and climbing the stairway to ecstasy.

Spirit Tools and Skills—Honoring the Sacredness of Sex

For me, sex is sacred for two reasons. First, because it produces life. Over the course of my professional career (and once as a mother), I've witnessed about 500 babies being born. Every time has reinforced my awe at sex's magical ability to create life. How can such a miracle be anything but sacred? Second, Eros is the primal life force. When we have sex, whether it's with others or ourselves, we are tapping into that root energy. We become connected to that universal Oneness—in other words, to the divine.

This section is premised on the notion that sex is a sacred, spiritual activity (which doesn't make it any less hot, wet and lusty!). You don't need to agree with this to benefit from what follows, though. If you're of a more secular or traditional religious bent, feel free to treat the exercises and rituals I describe as games or, alternatively, as structures that support accelerated learning. Whether or not you frame them as

Traditional Icon of
Divine Union, India

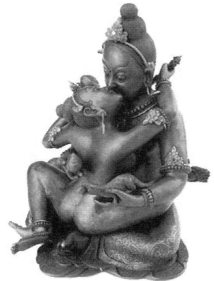

spiritual, these ideas and practices can add depth and richness to your relationship with yourself and others.

The Spirit Tools

SACRED INTENTION AND ATTITUDE are ways we hold things in our mind to keep them sacrosanct.

ALTARS AND SACRED SPACES are physical manifestations of our sacred intentions.

PRAYER, MEDITATION AND SACRED SOUND are ways to practice and help manifest our sacred intentions.

RITUAL AND CEREMONY help create sacred containers; they channel energy and matter in the service of our intentions.

"Let there be pleasure and ecstasy
on earth and let it begin with me."

ANNIE SPRINKLE

SACRED INTENTION AND ATTITUDE

Common parlance has it that we "hold" an intention. It's an interesting usage; what it tells us is that we create a container for it inside our mind where we can keep an eye on it and make sure it doesn't escape us.

We do this because we want to *manifest* the intention, and creating a container, if only a mental one, is a first step in that direction. It helps us take something invisible and begin the process of making it visible in the world—and that, when you think about it, is a pretty good definition of magic.

What makes an intention or attitude "sacred?" Because it involves our connection to Spirit.

ALTARS AND SACRED SPACES

One way to support our sacred intentions is by creating sacred spaces. When we do this, we're essentially taking the container that we erected inside our head and transferring it to physical space; we're mapping it onto the world. Sacred altars and erotic temples are how we keep a firm grip on our dreams and support our ongoing practice.

THE GODDESS GUIDE
Creating Your Magical Altar

You'll want to start by finding a space in your home for an assemblage of items that represent your sexuality to you. If you don't have a big enough space for a permanent altar, set it up on a tray. That way, you can move it to different places or put it away. This is also particularly useful if you aren't inclined to share it with people—your parents may not want to see that dildo on your altar (or anywhere, for that matter!).

Take some time beforehand to meditate on who you are currently as a sexual being and who you'd like to be. How would you make these invisible current and future aspects of yourself visible?

You might want to start with a piece of gorgeous cloth, perhaps red velvet or pink satin. Place something on your altar cloth that represents you, maybe a picture, a drawing or an animal totem. A traditional tantric altar would have a yoni-lingam on it representing the male and female principles. A typical pagan altar has items that signify water, fire, air and earth. You might want to include something that invokes Spirit in whatever form resonates with you. Do you want to call out your wild animal nature? Then put an image or representation of a wild animal. Are you trying to cultivate more sexual mindfulness? Perhaps a small mirror will remind you of that intention. If you're seeking a partner, put something on the altar that symbolizes the person you wish to call to you. If you have a sweetie, you might want to represent that person on the altar. (Voodoo dolls are probably not a good idea!)

Think of your altar as something that's always changing and evolving. When an item no longer resonates, remove it. Add new items as new intentions arise or as new ideas, projects, learnings and practices enter your life.

Take time as often as possible to sit at your altar. Meditate on your intentions. Repeat affirmations. Chant or sing sacred songs. Practice arousal skills or do orgasmic meditations there. Use your altar to focus on your goals and aspirations.

THE GODDESS GUIDE
Creating Your Perfect Erotic Temple

*D*o you have a special space in your home for sacred eroticism? No? Then let's create one. Ideally, we'd all have plenty of space and could dedicate a whole room to being a love-making temple. Most of us don't have that luxury, though. Don't let that stop you! Whether you use your current bedroom, a spare room or your living room, you can create a beautiful, luscious place to encounter the sexy Divine.

Step One: take time to envision what your perfect erotic temple would look like. Step Two: see how close you can come to making it real. Select which space in your home you'll use. If its sole purpose is as a sex space, it should be easy to put in mattresses, curtains, conveniently situated tables and erotically appropriate décor. Lots of pillows are always good.

If you're having one space do double-duty, give thought to how you can easily transition the space from its mundane to its sacred function and back again. It's easy to create soft lighting with candles or dim lamps, and you can get rid of any unsightly mess with a curtain or by tossing decorative throws over it. Keep computers, phones and televisions turned off and out of sight. Keep paperwork

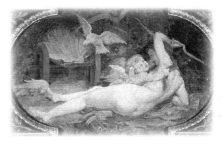

Paul Jacques-Aime Baudry—*Venus Playing with Cupid, c. 1860*

stashed away, too, unless you're one of the very small minority who finds bills erotic. Include your altar in your erotic temple. Living plants or fresh flowers always add beauty and life. You'll want to have plenty of lube handy, and also a convenient place for any toys.

Once you've got your space ready to your satisfaction, do a transition ritual to claim it as your sacred temple. Use incense or aromatherapy spritzers to cleanse the energy. Put on ecstatic music and consecrate the space in whatever manner works best for you. Welcome yourself to it! If you're sharing it with your lover (or lovers), welcome them as a priest or priestess would to their sacred space.

PRAYER, MEDITATION AND SACRED SOUND

As we saw in Chapter Nine, meditation helps us discipline our monkey-brain and learn to pay better attention. As such, it can help us become more aware of our mental, physical and emotional processes, both when we're having sex and at other times, too. But what about meditation makes it *spiritual*? This: by bringing meditative awareness to what we do, we pull back from the hustle and bustle of everyday awareness, and this distancing—dis-identification, in technical jargon—makes it easier for us to create a sacred space where it's easier to be more present and attuned.

"If the only prayer you said in your whole life was, "thank you," that would suffice."

MEISTER ECKHART

We saw earlier in this chapter that sound is one of our basic body skills, and that one of the things it does is create a sympathetic vibration. Sacred sound is the basic body skill of sound used for spiritual purposes, uttered with the intention of using this power of resonance to create or enrich a spiritual container, whether that be your room or your body. Anyone who's done sacred chanting, alone or in a group, knows how effective it can be.

Another way to use sound in the service of the sacred is through the use of prayer. Whether spoken, written, chanted or sung, words are a way to create sacred intention. When you speak holy affirmations, you form a verbal path to Spirit.

RITUAL AND CEREMONY

Rituals and ceremonies are formalized activities that help us access the sacred. They are effective because they are informed by the quite specific intention to open us to the divine, the mystical and the miraculous. Step by structured step, they act out that

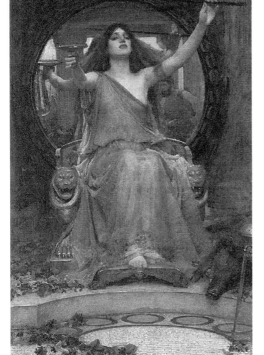

JOHN WILLIAM WATERHOUSE—*Circe Offering the Cup to Ulysses, c. 1880*

THE GODDESS GUIDE
Honor Your Sacred Sexual Self

*C*reate a sacred space in the ways we've already discussed. Be in your temple and have your altar nearby, along with whatever goodies you need for a solo-sex session. I strongly recommend having some lovely coconut oil handy.

Begin by setting an intention that reflects your desire for your self-sex to be sacred. Some suggestions: "I honor my sexual self," "I celebrate my pleasure," "I love my sexy body," "My yoni or lingam is sacred," "Sex is sacred play."

Now bring your focus to your breath, sound and pelvic muscle pumps. When you feel centered and present, start to touch yourself. (This is where the coconut oil comes in handy!) Start with your non-erogenous zones and work your way towards the sexier bits. Take your time and breathe, make sound and repeat your affirmations.

WHEN YOU'RE READY, bring your energy and focus to your genitals, showering them with love, touch, breath and positive words. Take as long as you'd like to bring your sexual energy up.

You may want to play with delaying your orgasm and circulating the energy. To do this, when you're close to coming, pause in your touch and do the following: draw the energy out of your genitals by breathing and sounding it up your spine, and then rolling it around in your head before allowing it to settle back down in your crotch. You may want to play with this circuit three or more times before you go into orgasmic release. When you are having your orgasm (or orgasms), repeat your affirmation (in a simplified form—your mind will be down in the brain-basement!) and dedicate the power and energy to your sacred parts, imagining your yoni or lingam suffused with light, love and bliss.

AFTER YOU'VE COME, gently hold your hands over your crotch and shower your parts with appreciation and honor. End by leaving a hand there and putting the other hand on your heart. Take three breaths, circulating sacred love within yourself.

intention, and in so doing make it easier for us to transfer those intentions from the mind-space to the physical "reality realm." They help create containers; they direct and channel energy and matter.

If you have an intention relating to your sexuality, meditation, sacred sound, ritual and ceremony are all great ways to accelerate the desired transformation.

We've now covered the four main set of skills—mind, heart, body and spirit. I encourage you to practice them regularly. The enchanted erosphere of sexual virtuosity awaits you!

THE GODDESS GUIDE
Sensual Self-Pleasure Ritual

Gather a variety of items to play with that resonate for you. Some recommendations: instruments or other items that make sound; objects or images of beauty; things that smell wonderful; an assortment of touchy-feely items; and tasty treats. Ideally, you will have a hand mirror present, along with some music that you can easily cue up. Light some candles or have the lights on dim.

You can do this ritual with or without self-sex play. I encourage you to try it both ways, or to start without the sex play and add it later. Have your sensual items and toys near at hand. Do whatever works for you to create a safe and sacred space.

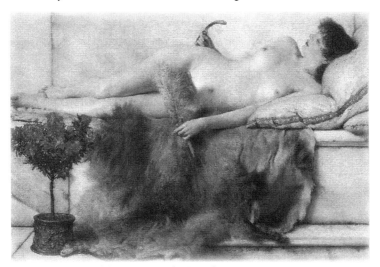

LAWRENCE ALMA-TADEMA—*In the Tepidarium, c. 1890*

I highly recommend trying this with your outer vision turned off. Close your eyes or put on a blindfold. Start with sound, either by playing with your sound toys or starting up some music. Tune your senses into the sound. Breathe it in. You can also sing, chant, hum or just play with your own ability to make sounds.

Now play with smells, amplifying the odors by deeply breathing them in and exhaling with purrs of pleasure. Next move on to feeding yourself, slowly savoring each bite, licking lusciously. Give yourself permission to sigh and moan and make other yummy sounds as you relish the delicious flavors in your mouth. Then move on to touch. Delight in your silky skin, tenderly stroke your own face, massage your feet or neck and generally explore the multitude of ways to touch and feel yourself. Rub fur on your belly, tickle yourself with a feather, scratch your back with a back scratcher, use a loofah on your legs or caress your inner arms with a piece of silk. Keep using your breath and sound as you play with touch.

If you're bringing this into the realm of the sexual, now start to stimulate your more erogenous areas. Fondle your breasts, squeeze your nipples, rub your rump, excite your equipment and pet your parts. Add your pelvic floor muscles to the game.

When you feel complete with this part of the ritual (orgasm optional), remove your blindfold, open your eyes and drink in beauty. Look in the mirror and see yourself shining back out. Delight in a gorgeous image. Gaze at a flower and be filled with awe at the glory of sight. Look out the window and take in the wonder of what you see. End with three or more conscious, deep, loving breaths, fully releasing each with an exuberant sound, while appreciating the gift of your senses and your inner tools for enhancing them.

CHAPTER ELEVEN

Energy Magic and Smart Slut Tricks

"Too much of a good thing can be wonderful."

MAE WEST

Do You Believe in (Energy) Magic?

WE'VE NOW REVIEWED YOUR FOUR MAIN TOOLS—the sexual skill sets of your mind, heart, body and spirit. Although it's convenient to treat them as if they were separate (and it's also true that, at one level, they are), they're also bound together by a common quality—energy.

We've touched on sexual energy throughout this book and played with it as well. Now let's consider an underlying truth: the real purpose of learning to play your instrument is not to become technically proficient—it's to be able to work with erotic energy so your orchestra creates amazing orgasmic improvisational symphonies.

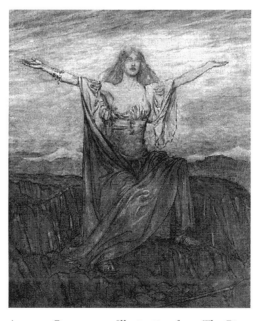

ARTHUR RACKHAM—*Illustration from The Ring*

We all know what sexual energy is. Birds know it, bees know it, even educated fleas know it. It's the force that impels life to makes life. It's the breathtaking swell of lust, the juice that makes us fall madly in love, the sizzle of romance and desire.

In hot new relationships, sexual energy sweeps us along with the unstoppable power of a stream swollen with spring rain. Often, this so-called new relationship energy fades once the flood ebbs and the freshness wears off. Partners sour on each other as the glow diminishes and they start seeing each other's faults and foibles. The realities of ordinary life—problem children and dirty dishes, declining parents and job stress, illness and errands—intrude. The chemical soup that sent us into that rushing river dissipates in the everyday swamp of the mundane world. Boredom takes over.

We can't make ourselves or our lives perfect, but we can keep our erotic energy alive, both over time and in individual encounters. Sexual energy isn't something entirely outside our control like a rainbow or a windstorm. It lives inside as well as around us, and we can learn to channel, build and ride it.

The Enchantment Gateway

Some of us have a greater natural aptitude for working with energy than others. Everyone can do it, though, and for many of us, it helps to be in an altered state—and, more specifically, the sort of altered state that heightens our awareness of subtle realms. As it happens, sexual arousal is precisely this sort of altered state! Which means, conveniently, that when you're turned on, it's easier to sense and work with sexual energy. Gee, you'd almost think God(dess) intended it that way!

Playing consciously with sexual energy doesn't just happen, though. It's an ability we must cultivate.

We can work with sexual energy alone or with a partner. When you do it by yourself, you go into a *solo trance*. Once there, you play with your own internal erotic circuits. You give and you get, being both yang initiator (*you* have to initiate sex with yourself!) and yin receiver. All your attention and awareness are focused inward (while you may have imaginary playmates, they always do exactly what you want right when you want it!). You're in your own world on your private arousal journey.

When we play duets (or trios or quartets or . . .), we're collaborating to make erotic music. There are two possible avenues for this shared journey. A *parallel trance* occurs when we're in a self-trance, and so is our partner. This means that energetically, we spend much of our time caught up in our own inner experience, even though we're in physical contact with the other person.

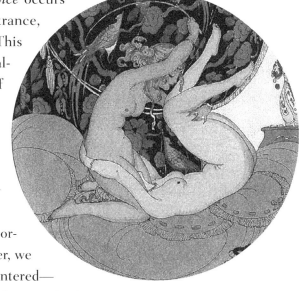

Needless to say, in order to be a good partner, we can't be totally self-centered— we need to attend to whoever else is there (it's only polite!). Partners in solo trance

Gerda Wegener, c. 1920

often wind up taking turns. I attend to your arousal trance, you attend to mine and so on, with our energy and attention ping-ponging back and forth. Everyone, including sexual virtuosos, sometimes plays this way.

There's nothing wrong with this pattern, although sometimes the more elusive feminine yin arousal is neglected when a yang partner's more urgent arousal energy claims center stage. But even when the alternating attention of the parallel trance is working, there's a better way to go on an erotic energy trip with a partner.

A *connected trance* brings partners into profound attunement. When partners share an erotic trance, not only are they sharing the same sexual field with each other (which, of course, happens to some extent whenever people have sex), but they're also having the identical experience of that energy's subtle and powerful flows. Their energy circuits are literally linked. It's as if the lovers are sharing an invisible musical score—*The Opus of Sexual Energy*—and they're playing in perfect time with each other. It's a sexually telepathic state, and it can feel miraculous when it happens.

"I trust all joy."

THEODORE ROETHKE

It's not, though. Becoming energetically attuned in a shared trance is an acquired skill we can learn through training and practice. And, of course, as with all things sexual, it starts with learning to make your own instrument sing.

The Sexual Energy eXperience (S.E.X.)

We experience sexual energy through the filter of who we are, and since we're all different, our experiences vary. There is one overarching commonality, though: people always report a sense of movement. Whatever else it might be, sexual energy isn't static. Beyond that, individual variability takes over:

- Some people experience sexual energy as moving heat, like a flow of molten lava or a torrent of hot water.

- Others feel vibrations pulsing through them.

- Some see light and colors swirling.

- People sometimes report sounds thrumming and beating rhythms inside them.

- Some feel sensations tingling and awakening various body parts.

- Yet others report multiple sensations that mutate as the energy awakens, builds and surges about.

Whatever you're feeling, I encourage you to trust the experience. If you feel something happening, it is.

The Three Laws of Sexual Energy

Like all natural forces, sexual energy is governed by certain immutable laws. We cannot alter these realities any more than we can levitate. We have to understand and work within them.

Yin and Yang

The first truth about sexual energy is a familiar one: it participates in the grand dance of yin and yang. To work effectively with sexual energy, you need to call on both qualities. You need to be able to surrender to sexual energy (yin) while also actively directing it (yang). Because sexual energy is very fluid, you can't force it, only channel the flow—you can't push the river, as the saying goes.

That's not enough, though. You also need to be actively (though subtly) yang. You have to be like the archetypal Magician, using your attention and intention to call forth the energy with your special skills and spells.

Hot, Hot, Hot

The second truth is that sexual energy is fiery. To make a fire, you need three ingredients—fuel, oxygen and heat.

The *fuel* for sexual energy is the associated emotions of attraction, desire and pure old animal lust. Strong positive feelings such as love, caring and appreciation can also provide the spark. Other powerful emotions like anger and humiliation are a turn-on for some, too.

> *"Only the united heat of sex and heart together can create ecstasy."*
>
> ANAIS NIN

Relief can also rev things up. If this doesn't seem intuitively obvious to you, think about make-up sex—almost breaking up is one of the great aphrodisiacs.

Surface appearances are another potent fuel. This is partly evolutionary—we are programmed to equate physical attractiveness with desirable genes—and partly cultural—the mainstream media peddle youth and beauty with the 24/7 insatiability of a cartoon nymphomaniac.

This type of fuel tends to run out fast, one reason celebrity marriages have a high turnover rate. When people connect at a deeper and more authentic level, it produces a much more enduring fire.

Finally, any discussion of erotic fuels would be incomplete without a mention of boredom—not because it helps heat things up, but because it does the opposite. Boredom is to arousal as anti-matter is to matter. It's the universal fire extinguisher.

The *oxygen* is supplied by our breath. Just as we blow on a fire to make it burn hotter, we can build arousal by breathing into it. In fact, this little bit of erotic know-how—that arousal is ramped up by breath—is the secret sauce that puts the sizzle in Lauren Bacall's famous line to Humphrey Bogart in the film *To Have and Have Not*: "You know how to whistle, don't you, Steve? You just put your lips together and . . . *blow*."

The heat for sexual energy is provided by the wonderful mammalian hot-blooded furnace of our body. Most female mammals need to be fertile to go into "heat" and be receptive to mating. We human females, on the other hand, can go into heat anytime we want (especially when we use both hands!).

Men and women alike also have a handy tool in our mind—our imaginations, which can provide an unlimited supply of highly combustible fuel, customized to the exact specifications of our engine.

YOU CAN'T PUSH THE RIVER, BUT YOU CAN DAM IT UP

The third law is that sexual energy can be blocked or dammed, especially by negative feelings like anger, hurt and resentment. Fear and its less operatic cousin, anxiety, are especially effective at blocking sexual energy. The hormones that are released during these states are directly antithetical to the ones that support the shift into the trance of sexual arousal.

> *"If you obey all the rules, you miss all the fun."*
>
> KATHARINE HEPBURN

Our inhibitions are another energy blocker. Some of these are outside our awareness, either because they're buried deep in our unconscious or because they're so endemic to our culture as to be virtually invisible. There are also the inhibitions that we're well aware of. Shaming inner voices, limiting gender roles and low-self esteem are just a few of the influences that can block the free flow of sexual energy.

Blocks can be dismantled, of course. If they're unconscious, they can be brought into awareness, and once they've been made conscious, we can work with them to diminish or eliminate their impact on our lives.

Making It Happen

Three basic steps are involved in working with sexual energy. You need to:

- Have faith in its existence, not merely as a theoretical construct but as something you can move and shape. Ya gotta believe it to perceive it!

- Allow yourself to release your inhibitions and go into an altered state.

- Use your mind, body, heart and spirit skills.

As I've said, you've already been playing with your erotic energy when you worked with your tools, especially breath, sound, and motion. What we're adding to the mix here is two things—first, using your inner vision to see the energy pathways, and second, using your intention to work with and move that energy.

ANCIENT MODELS

Due to our Western culture's mechanistic paradigm, it can be difficult to be sure that what you imagine is really so. It's hard to trust our intuition, especially if it's been denigrated and denied.

Fortunately, we're not alone in wanting to understand and master energy systems. Over the course of millennia, many cultures have developed maps that portray how energy concentrates and circulates in the body.

Drawing from these wells of ancient wisdom, I recommend three simple schemes to play with. In the first, which is drawn from tantra, there is a central channel that forms a hollow pipe running right up through the center of your body (or, alternatively, up your spinal cord). One end is in your crotch and the other is at your mouth or the top of your head, or both. (This was the basis for the "Opening the Tube" visualization exercise in the last chapter.)

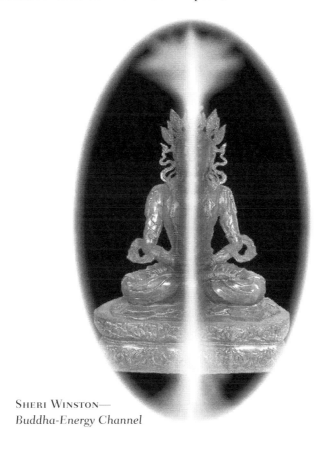

SHERI WINSTON—
Buddha-Energy Channel

The Taoist sexual wisdom tradition describes a somewhat different circuit, the "microcosmic orbit." In this model, a current runs down the front of your belly, around your bottom, up your back, through your head and back down your front to your belly.

Pumping the Microcosmic Orbit

Our pelvic powerhouse is one of our main sites for circulating sexual energy through our body and into our surrounding field. The more you learn to enhance this natural conduit, the stronger and more powerfully you'll be able to run energy through it.

Visualize the energy starting in your belly. Draw it to down to your crotch, then into your sacrum. Bring it up the spine, swirl it around in your head, touch your tongue to the roof of your mouth, and let it flow down the front and come to rest in your solar plexus.

Now repeat, using your inhaled breath to pull the energy up your spine. This time, hold your breath while you swirl it in your head, then exhale it down your front. Repeat.

After you've got the basics down, try adding sound to your exhale. Explore different types of sound to find out what most supports the energy flow.

Now play with adding your pelvic floor muscles to the game. Try pulling up with your pelvic muscles on the inhale, holding them as you swirl energy in your head, and releasing your bottom on the exhale.

With each new experience, note what happens. Enjoy. And if the energy wave starts to really move, jump on and ride it!

The third model that's particularly useful is the chakra system of traditional India, which is widely used in modern tantra and yoga. (Chakra is a Sanskrit word meaning wheel or vortex.) The best-known chakra system uses seven energy vortexes, although some have more and some have less.

The chakra system helps us understand where energy concentrates in our bodies, and for what purpose. The chakras operate like pumps or valves, regulating our flow of energy and key aspects of our consciousness. They primarily interact with the physical body through the endocrine and nervous systems. Each has a physical location, emotional and energetic aspects, and is also associated with a color, a sound, a sense, an element, an endocrine gland, a specific group of nerves, body parts, functions and systems.

The Seven-Vortex Chakra System

Here is a brief overview of the chakra system that is best known in western countries:

CROWN CHAKRA

Location: Top of the head

Color: Violet or white

Associations: Cosmic and divine energy. Oneness with the universe. Nirvana.

THIRD EYE or BROW CHAKRA

Location: Center of forehead

Color: Indigo

Associations: Mind. Brain. Intuition. Intellect. Knowledge. Wisdom.

THROAT CHAKRA

Location: Base of the throat

Color: Sky blue

Associations: Communication. Authentic expression. Trust.

HEART CHAKRA

Location: Center of the chest

Color: Emerald green

Associations: Love in all forms— romantic, passionate, familial, patriotic, friendly.

SOLAR PLEXUS CHAKRA

Location: Solar plexus

Color: Yellow

Associations: Personal power. Vitality. Control. Freedom.

LOWER BELLY or SEX CHAKRA

Location: Genitals, Pelvis

Color: Orange

Associations: Sex. Reproduction. Creativity. Intimate Relationships. Survival of the Species.

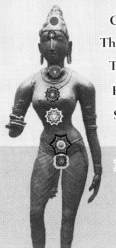

Crown

Third Eye

Throat

Heart

Solar

Sex

Root

ROOT or PERINEUM CHAKRA

Location: The perineum

Color: Red

Associations: Birth. Life. Personal Survival. Safety. Security. Groundedness. Earth connection.

Chakra Charging Meditation Practice

Create a sacred space for this, or use the one you've created. Make sure you won't be interrupted by ringing phones or other distractions. Put on music if you'd like.

Get in a comfortable position. You can lie on your back with your knees up and feet flat on the floor. You can sit with your spine straight in a relaxed upright position. Or, you can stand with your feet shoulder-width apart and your knees loose and unlocked.

Close your eyes. Start by taking a few deep centering breaths, then exhaling with an audible sigh, sound or tone. Now begin to focus on your perineum and your root chakra. As you inhale, imagine earth energy flowing up into your first chakra. As you exhale with sound, imagine a root that extends from your bottom down into the earth. Inhale and feel energy flowing like sap up into your perineal center. Exhale with sound and feel your connection to the earth growing deeper. After you feel a strong connection, begin to breathe in and out with your focus staying on the root chakra. Imagine a red ball of energy that swirls and pulses with each breath. Increase the pace of your breathing and allow your sound to grow as well. Keep going until your root chakra feels like it's full of energy and secure in its connection to the earth.

Now, slow your breath and bring your attention up to your sex chakra, which includes your genitals and the pelvic bowl. Imagine a vortex of orange light that suffuses the area with each breath. Continue to inhale into your second chakra and exhale with a sound. Increase the depth and pace of your breathing until your pelvis feels filled with hot orange energy.

Slow your breath again and bring your attention to your solar plexus. Imagine yellow sunlight streaming in with your inhale and radiating out with your exhale. Continue to use your sound. Increase the intensity of the breath until your third chakra feels filled with power and vitality.

Quiet your breath again and draw your awareness up into your heart chakra. Imagine a green shining light suffusing you as you inhale and receive love. Exhale with sound and give love out. Increase the pace until you feel that you are love, Beloved and lover all at once.

*O*nce more, allow your breath to quiet and bring your energy and attention up to your throat chakra. See brilliant sky-blue light pour in as you inhale, and see it radiate out as you release your breath with beautiful sound. Again, pick up the pace, breathing deeply and quickly until your throat is full of singing and your voice shines fully out.

Slow your breath again and bring your attention up to your third eye, the sixth chakra, center of intuition and intellect. Imagine your breath moving in and out through your opened forehead. Breathe more deeply and feel your inner eye open wide, with brilliant violet light streaming in and out.

Slow your breathing again and bring your awareness to the top center of your head, your crown chakra. Imagine it dilating, opening up to connect to a flow of divine white light energy from above. Increase the pace of the breath and feel the streaming power entering you from above.

Now, send your breath and sound all the way up and down your inner channel, connecting at the bottom with embodied earth energy and at the top with the energy of disembodied spirit consciousness. Stay in this place, breathing the connection up and down, allowing the sensation and experience to fill and flow through you.

When you feel utterly full of the flow, imagine it showering out from the top of your head, cascading like a prismatic fountain around you. Enjoy feeling surrounded, caressed, safe, abundant and ecstatic within the breath of the sacred universe.

When you're ready, allow the breath to slow and the glow to settle. Take a few moments to sit peacefully, quietly appreciating yourself, your life and your capacity for joy.

End with a prayer of gratitude.

There are many other models of energy flow in addition to the three I've discussed. For instance, another map from the tantric traditions identifies three channels—a central channel and lateral ones on either side of the body. Another map is based on the meridians of traditional Chinese medicine, which are used in the science and art of acupuncture.

Collectively, these models are a living reminder that people have been dancing with energy for millennia. While it's true that different cultures recognized different patterns, this shouldn't be taken as evidence that they're invalid. For one thing, there's enormous overlap among them. For another, there is increasing empirical evidence that they have merit. To take just one example, acupuncture has been shown to be effective for surgical anesthesia.

I invite you to try out these models, using your inner vision to guide you. The more you see the energy flowing, the more you will actually experience it. Find out what works for you: it may be one model, it may be more than one in combination, and it may be a spin-off you discover on your own.

Smart Slut Tricks

Now that you know more about your energy systems, let's learn how you can put them to great use, specifically by developing some advanced sex skills. I call them "smart slut tricks" because it takes practice to develop these abilities, and a dedicated slut would presumably like nothing better than to spend hours of happy time honing her talents. (As noted earlier, I use "slut" to mean anyone, man or woman, who has a healthy, uninhibited attitude toward sex. In my book, this is a very good thing, and I hope it is in yours, too.)

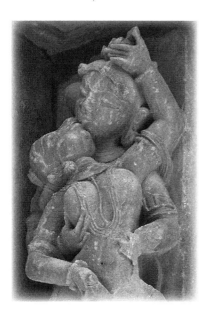

Chitragupta Temple, India

PATHWAYS TO PLEASURE

Would you like to be able to have an orgasm from having your nipples stimulated or your neck licked? Or perhaps from having your earlobe nibbled on?

How about being able to come while you're talking on the phone with your sweetie, on the count of three— without touching yourself? (And I mean a real orgasm, not the phony— or, rather, phone-y—pay-by-the-minute sort!)

---

* As for "smart slut tricks," that plays off "stupid pet tricks," a term some of you may recall from David Letterman's early days. I don't expect we'll be seeing any 'smart sluts' on late night shows to demonstrate these advanced skills. One can always hope, though.

Would you like to be able to climax, repeatedly, when you're going down on your partner and your hands are, shall we say, otherwise occupied?

If these things sound like fun to you, read on. I can't promise that you'll be able to do them all by the time you've finished reading this book, but at least you'll know how to learn them.

Play and Practice
Developing Orgasmic Proficiency

Before you can master these advanced skills, you need to be orgasmically proficient. Here are the basics of what you need to know to do this:

- HONOR WHERE YOU ARE in your learning journey. Wherever you are, it's totally okay, and since this is all learnable stuff, there's no need to despair.

- MAKE A PERSONAL COMMITMENT to expand your arousal paths— and to do it on your own, not with a partner. You want to make it easy on yourself, and partnered sex presents a separate set of issues and challenges. Save that for later.

- PRACTICE YOUR BASICS—a lot! Get really good at using your triad of breath, sound and movement to pump up your sexual energy. Ideally, you'll get to the point where you automatically use your basic toolkit when you're having sex, whether it's solo or partnered.

- PLAY WITH YOUR TOYS. For many women, the easiest path to orgasm involves the use of an additional tool—a vibrator. A hand-held shower massager can also do the trick. Try out different toys and find one or several that you like. Incorporate using your toy into your solo-sex play, along with your personal inner toolkit. (Of course, taking matters into your own hot little hands is fine, too! Use whatever works for you.)

- PLAY AND PRACTICE WITHOUT AN AGENDA other than exploring your pleasure. Generally speaking, plenty of practice without pressure will yield orgasmic results. When you can travel to your climactic destination every time, you've developed *orgasmic proficiency.*

"Some men know that a light touch of the tongue, running from a woman's toes to her ears, lingering in the softest way possible in various places in between, given often enough and sincerely enough, would add immeasurably to world peace."

MARIANNE WILLIAMSON

YOUR PERSONAL PATHS

Your erotic journey began when you first explored your capacity for sexual pleasure. Sooner or later, most of us stumbled on a path that took us to orgasm—and we saw that it was good! So good, in fact, that we went back often, usually following the same path that got us there the first time.

Familiar pathways are a fine and useful thing. An established trail reliably and quickly gets you where you want to go. They have a downside, though. When you use the same path over and over again, it can become a rut, eventually eroding into a deep trench. It can become the only way, instead of one of many possible ways to go.

We can teach ourselves to expand our network of trails by using a simple animal-training technique. (Yup, lions and tigers and pussies, oh my!)

After all, if Pavlov could get a dog to salivate when he rang a bell by associating the ting-a-ling with scrumptious snacks, you can learn to come by associating arousal and orgasm with . . . anything you want. You learn smart slut tricks by cross-training your brain.

THE ROAD TO ORGASMIC ABUNDANCE

You start by taking your usual path to pleasure. Let's say you take your vibrator out and start playing with your clit. Your brain knows where this is headed and thinks, in the non-verbal, gray-matter way brains think: "I know this path—let's go!" Then, at the same time you're buzzing away, you add a new activity to your usual one, such as stimulating your nipples. Soon your brain starts connecting the two: "Nipples and clit together, oh boy, that means an orgasmic treat!" You do this for a while until your brain has carved out a new neural pathway. Now you have two parallel paths: one equates clitoral play with orgasm and the other associates nipple stimulation with orgasm. Here's where the trick comes in: because the brain experiences them as producing the same result—orgasm—it starts viewing them as interchangeable.

After you've got both trails laid down, you go on to the next level of training. Now, you start as before, but intermittently stop using the vibrator and keep on keeping on with your nipples. Employ your toolkit, especially breath, sound, pelvic floor pumping and your imagination to keep your arousal trance heading up the stairs. Return your vibrator to your clit whenever you need to continue your journey to orgasm.

The final level of training happens at high-level arousal. Use both paths, but stop the clitoral stimulation when you're almost coming, and—you guessed it—pulse, breathe, imagine and send your sound and energy down into your crotch and … what happens? Your body-mind is already hurtling down the orgasmic highway, and it just keeps going (and coming). Now that it believes nipple stimulation is as effective an orgasmic strategy as clit-play, what's a brain to do but go, "Yes! Yes! Ohmigod, yes!"

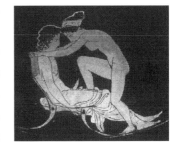

Greece, 420 BC

You can use this technique to teach yourself every manner of sex skill. And please note: the parallel-track training method isn't only for advanced students—you can also use it for more basic skills.* You can learn how to:

- Have an orgasm if you've never had one before.

- Discover your reliable path to orgasm if you don't have one.

- Expand your pathways to orgasm, including orgasm with intercourse (which is, by far, the best way to enjoy penetration!).

- Have simultaneous orgasm. (You'll need a partner for that, of course.)

- Do smart slut tricks such as coming from non-genital stimulation—the only limit here is your imagination.

Whether it's a relatively basic skill or a super-duper smart slut trick, the process is simple: you decide what you want to do, and go ahead and learn it. Whatever the level, the basic learning strategy is the same— cross-train your brain.

---

* Guys, this technique isn't just for women. You can use it too, for instance, to learn to have non-ejaculatory energy orgasms.

Play and Practice
ExpandingYour Orgasmic Pathways

Let's say you're a woman who can only have orgasms by using a vibrator on your clit when you're alone, and you'd like to develop pathways that don't require electronic assistance.

Begin by playing with yourself in your usual way. Get yourself to a medium or high level of arousal.

Intermittently take away your vibrator and use your hand instead, while staying attuned to your arousal level. Meanwhile, keep using your inner arousal toolkit of breath, sound and pelvic floor movements (you've been practicing that, right?). Also use your imagination, visualizing your clit vibrating or being gently sucked or whatever turns you on.

As soon as you notice your arousal dropping down, put your vibrator back on your clitoris. Return to your familiar arousal trail as often as you need to. (Don't let this get you down: it's all part of the learning process.) Keep going, using your vibrator as much as you need to, but continuing to build out a new path by removing that form of stimulation and using different ones. Over time, you'll find that you need to use your vibrator less and less as using your hand becomes an established pathway to orgasm.

Now, if your batteries die, it won't be a disaster!

GETTING OFF WHILE GETTING THEM OFF

Here's an example of a much-appreciated smart slut trick you can learn: you can come by giving head. That's right, you can get off by going down!

You'll have to master some preliminaries first, though. To start with, you'll need to really, really like genitals—how they look, smell, taste and feel. This may require you to reprogram negative beliefs. If so, I encourage you to do that important work.

Teach yourself to delight in dining at the Y or swallowing the sacred scepter (or both). Learn to love the feel of the lingam or yoni in your mouth, against your lips and under your tongue. Your mouth is getting stimulated every time it's in contact, so pay attention to how wonderfully erotic those sensations are. Your mouth is an extremely sensitive erogenous zone. If you like kissing, then using your lips and tongue to give pleasure can also be pleasurable. Take time to use your entire oral orifice to explore, play with and discover your partner's equipment. Genitalia are beautiful, sweet, savory and sexy. Delight in the contours, the smooth and the furry textures, the many little sweet spots and the fact that whatever you're doing is driving your partner wild.

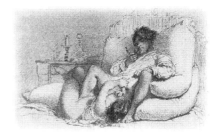

Once you're totally grooving on the activity, it's time to fool your brain. Play with yourself while you're going down on him or her. When you're on the verge of coming, take away the direct stimulus and keep nuzzling,

MIHALY ZICHY—*Making Love, c. 1890*

licking, slurping or whatever yummy thing you're doing. Repeat until the connection between going down and your own arousal is hardwired in your brain. Eventually, the hot connection between your mouth and your partner's genitals will be enough to send you over the top.

Play and Practice
A Super-Advanced Smart Slut Trick— The Deep Throat-gasm

Coming from deep-throating your partner . . . it sounds like a porn fantasy, right? And it is—but it's also a learnable skill.

Employing your basic toolkit of breath, sound, movement and touch, play with yourself in whatever way works, while also going down on your lover. Time things so you bring yourself to orgasm precisely when you take him into your throat. Repeat, and repeat again, until your brain has come, so to speak, to associate "cock in throat" with "orgasm." (Your sweetie won't object, I promise you!)

Now, deep-throat him while you're at the "I'm almost coming" state of arousal—and remove whatever you've been using to stimulate your genitals directly. That gullible brain of yours will go, "Oh boy, cock in throat, that means I should come!," and the predictable fireworks will follow.[1*]

---

* Clearly, you need to know how to perform deep throat before you can learn to climax from it. It's a learned skill—anyone can do it. While I won't be teaching the technique in this book, here's a tip: it's most easily done at high arousal. Remember that your upper and lower parts are connected, so when your mouth and throat are soft and open, your yoni is too—and vice-versa! It's much easier to take something large down your throat when your pussy is puffy and open.

One final thought: don't expect to learn these skills overnight. The brain can be fooled, but tricking (I mean training) it takes time. Stay with it, and enjoy the practice!

The Fountain of the Goddess—The Learnable Art of Female Ejaculation

Fifteen years ago, I didn't know about female ejaculation. No one had mentioned it during my many years of medical training or in my studies in the edgier realms of alternative healing. When I first heard about it, I dismissed it as yet another porn myth that creates an impossible standard for women.

"Graze on my lips; and if those hills be dry, stray lower, where the pleasant fountains lie."
WILLIAM SHAKESPEARE

Then I started to meet women who squirted. I became a believer that it was possible although, at the time, I assumed only a small number of unusual women had this mysterious ability. Once I got it that female ejaculation was real, I still didn't realize that it was a skill that could be acquired until I met women who had learned how to do it. Well, I figured if they could learn to gush, so could I—and I did! And so can you.

I now know that all women can learn to ejaculate. To become a gushing goddess, you need two things—an accurate understanding of the physiology and the associated processes, and the commitment to practice the relevant basic and advanced skills.

You already have all the necessary equipment.

THE AMRITA ELIXIR

What the ancient texts refer to as amrita comes out of the same hole that urine does. This causes a lot of people, assuming some who should know better (like doctors), to assume it's pee. It's not. For one thing, the smell is different: female ejacu-

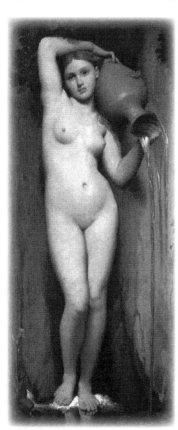

late smells lightly musky like fresh sea water.* Also, while it can emerge in a stream like urine, it often doesn't. It can issue in small trickles or sizable gushes, and it can also spout out like a geyser. This, too, varies from woman to woman, and for individual shejaculators as well—sometimes the same woman will trickle a few drops one day and the next day be Old Faithful.

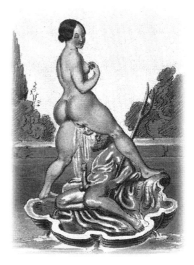

PETER FENDI—*The Fountain*

Nor is it vaginal lubrication. It's watery and not slippery, and it doesn't come out of the vagina.

When women ejaculate, it often but not always accompanies their orgasm. Whether it happens with or without a climax, it feels fabulous. Shejaculators usually find it to be an emotionally profound as well as physically feel-good experience.

WHERE DOES ALL THAT LIQUID COME FROM?

As we saw in Chapter Seven, the erectile tissue of the urethral sponge is composed of capillaries, which are blood vessels whose wall is only one cell thick. The paraurethral glands are composed of a multitude of networks of tiny tubules like the hair roots on a plant, which are enmeshed in the urethral erectile tissue. The wall of these microtubules is also one cell thick. What this means is that the watery part of our blood, called serum, can easily diffuse across the capillary membrane and enter the tubules of the gland. There, it mixes with the glands' secretions and becomes amrita.

When squirting time arrives, the ejaculate is emitted through the thirty tiny openings that connect the gland to the urethral canal, as well as through the two larger openings near the exit of the urethra. The fluid then flows down the urethra and emerges in varying amounts from the urethral opening. Since the source of the fluid is blood serum and the process of fluid diffusion is almost instantaneous, women can make large amounts of amrita and keep on doing so. This process is similar to how nursing mothers make breast milk, which can also be produced instantly and in copious amounts.

---

* The scent varies from woman to woman, just like our body odor and vaginal musk. It also varies depending on where a woman is in her fertility cycle.

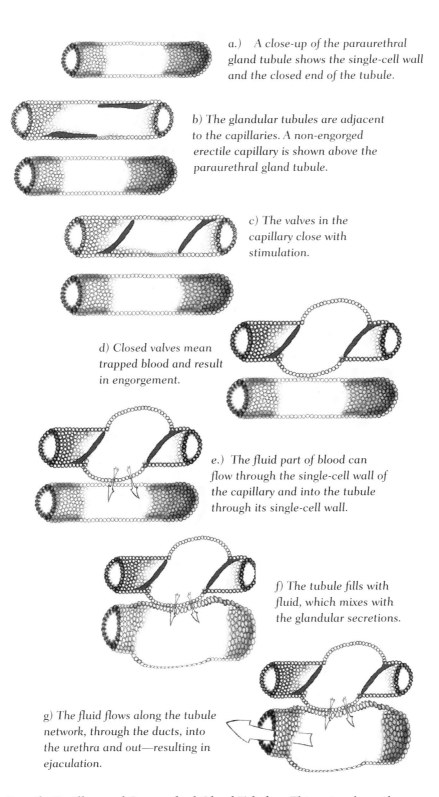

a.) A close-up of the paraurethral gland tubule shows the single-cell wall and the closed end of the tubule.

b) The glandular tubules are adjacent to the capillaries. A non-engorged erectile capillary is shown above the paraurethral gland tubule.

c) The valves in the capillary close with stimulation.

d) Closed valves mean trapped blood and result in engorgement.

e.) The fluid part of blood can flow through the single-cell wall of the capillary and into the tubule through its single-cell wall.

f) The tubule fills with fluid, which mixes with the glandular secretions.

g) The fluid flows along the tubule network, through the ducts, into the urethra and out—resulting in ejaculation.

Erectile Capillary and Paraurethral Gland Tubule— This series shows the process of fluid flow from the circulatory system via the erectile capillaries into the tubules of the paraurethral gland and then out. This produces the no-longer mysterious sacred amrita, also known as female ejaculate.

CALLING FORTH THE FOUNTAIN

For many women, the experience of ejaculation usually results from prolonged stimulation of the urethral sponge, often with multiple orgasms. This spongy area responds best to firm rhythmical pulling, rubbing and thrusting motions. Toys specifically designed for g-spot stimulation are especially useful as it's hard to rub your own urethral sponge with your own hand. If someone else is providing this service, fingers do a better job of directly stimulating the area than the cock, at least to start with.

This is an advanced skill that requires basic orgasmic ability along with proficiency in the use of your essential toolkit. As with many new skills, I recommend learning this with yourself before attempting it with a partner. Either way, it's best to be laid-back about this. Putting pressure on yourself to succeed will only get in the way. Have fun practicing and one day you'll be rewarded by the elixir's pouring forth. Like most sexual responses, it can be encouraged but not forced.

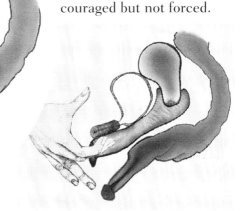

a) Side View. The urethral sponge and the adjacent structures.

b) Fingers stimulating the urethral sponge.

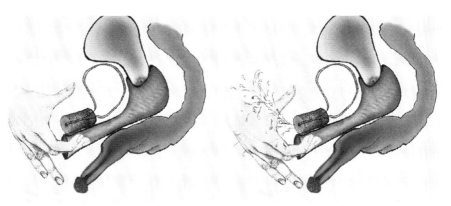

c) The sponge swells (and uterus rises).　　d) Squirting!

Play and Practice
A Squirting Primer

Start by preparing a puddle-proof space. Put down towels on top of waterproof pads. (The kinds used for toddler toilet-training are great!)

Have ample water nearby to stay well hydrated. Using bendy straws means that you don't have to sit up or change position to get frequent drinks.

Have your favorite toys at hand if you'll be using them. There are now a wide variety of g-spotter toys out there. And, of course, have plenty of your favorite lube.

Start with an empty bladder to decrease the worry that what comes out is pee.

Use your easiest pathways to become aroused. Take lots of time getting your whole arousal network engorged. You may wish to start by having a "regular" orgasm in your usual way.

Then use lots of firm rhythmic stimulation to the "goddess sponge" until you feel it swell. It should feel almost squishy. As orgasm approaches, bear down with your belly and pelvic muscles, opening and pushing out. Allow your mouth and throat to be open. too. Make big, deep, low-pitched open-mouthed sounds. As you ride the wave of your orgasm, continue to stimulate yourself, push and sound again, release, and let go. Repeat.

Try different positions. Experiment with various types of stimulation. Explore different toys. Try playing with your breathing patterns and sounds. Enjoy your orgasms, whether you squirt or not. One day, you will!

Owning It

We've now come to the end of your personal guided tour. (There is one additional side trip you may want to make, to a short last chapter especially directed toward men—although, of course, women are also welcome!)

I invite you to go play with your sexual energy . . . *a lot!* Learn to fully utilize your inner toolkit and play your instrument with skill and beauty. Practice and practice and practice some more! Have fun!

Remember this, though: there is no one correct path, no exact speed, no required destination.

Please also bear in mind that tools and techniques, no matter how useful, are not an end in themselves. Skill, enthusiasm and expertise can go a long way toward making you a sexual adept, but that is not true mastery. Ultimately, becoming an erotic virtuoso requires you to discover and tap into your own awesome erotic energy and power.

"Each morning we are born again. What we do today is what matters most."

BUDDHA

I wrote this book because I am committed to helping you and others revision what sex is and can be. You can choose to be a deeply sexual, whole and free person. You can choose to love sex, your body and your wonderful succulent self. If my experience is any measure, it can take years of reprogramming to make these choices and reclaim these qualities. Pay no heed to what's been laid down for you about what "good girls" do or don't do. Be your own authority! Ultimately, you are your own beautiful ongoing experiment in how to live a juicy life.

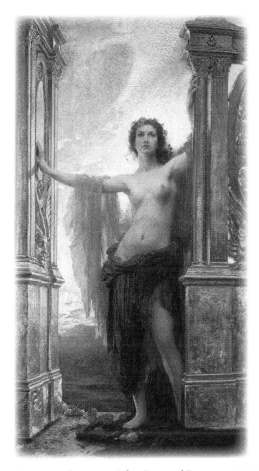

HERBERT DRAPER—*The Gates of Dawn, c. 1880*

I hope you've enjoyed this journey of discovery and exploration. More importantly, though, I hope you've been introduced to your erotic potential in a way that empowers you to keep travelling the road of conscious learning. Ecstasy, pleasure and delight in your sexuality are your birthright. Claim them! Your sexuality is your personal manifestation of the universal life force. Celebrate it!

So, in the end, this book isn't really ending, it's just beginning. If I've been at all successful in what I set out to do, I've planted a seed in you: I've empowered you to discover your own ecstatic gateway. I've provided many maps, but the real path is inside you. Where you go from here is up to you.

Blessings on your journey!

"Today, like every other day,
we wake up empty and frightened.
Don't open the door to the study
and begin reading. Take down a
musical instrument. Let the beauty
we love be what we do. There
are hundreds of ways to
kneel and kiss the ground."

RUMI

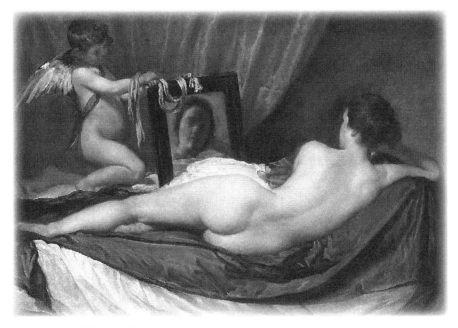

Velazquez—*The Rokeby Venus, c. 1640*

CHAPTER TWELVE

The Easy Girl's Guide to Making It Easy for Guys

"Some men spend a lifetime in an attempt to comprehend the complexities of women. Others preoccupy themselves with somewhat simpler tasks, such as understanding the theory of relativity!"

ALBERT EINSTEIN

It's Time for a Quickie!

In the pages that follow, I provide a "clit notes" version of pretty much everything you need to know to make the woman (or women) in your life very happy.

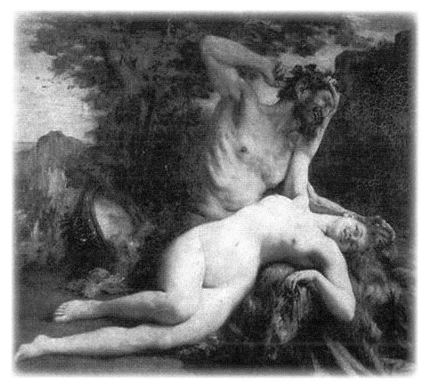

HENRI GERVEX—*Satyr and Nymph, c. 1920*

Your Lover-in-a-Box Kit, on a Count of Five

THE FIVE THINGS YOU NEED TO KNOW ABOUT WOMEN

1. Women are really, really different from you. Here's a good working guideline for you: whatever you'd want done to yourself, assume she wants the opposite. It's as if women inhabit a Bizarro World where everything is backwards. You'd like her to grab your cock as soon as possible, right? Well, applying the Bizarro Principle, that means she wants you to get to her crotch after you've taken lots of time warming up the rest of her.

2. More than anything, she wants to feel connected. She wants to talk and touch, to listen and share. Attention and presence create the context of affinity and attachment she craves.

3. She needs to feel safe in order to open and receive, and then to get turned on and orgasmic. If you try to barge in before she's ready, it will backfire on you. At best, you'll have to take three giant steps backwards. At worst, she'll Just Say No, this time or forever.

4. Now for the good news: when she does feel safe and connected, that's when she's most likely to want to have sex with you. That trusting connection will allow her to open way up!

5. Feminine flowers need sun and water to bloom—so shower her with appreciation, admiration, compliments and other positive yumminess. Give the woman what she wants and she'll blossom.

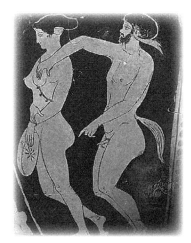

"Women speak two languages— one of which is verbal."

WILLIAM SHAKESPEARE

Ancient Greece—Satyr Caressing a Maenad

THE TOP FIVE MISTAKES GUYS MAKE WITH WOMEN

1. You don't attend to her body language and subtle signals.

2. You're clumsy, unsubtle and rough—too much poking, pounding, pushing, grabbing and groping.

3. You go to her genitals way too fast, diving into her crevices before she's warmed up enough. The result: she clams up—and maybe tosses you into that mental file cabinet where she keeps the negative stereotypes about guys she's been compiling over the years.

4. Having gotten to her genitals too soon, you make it even worse by attempting premature penetration. If she isn't highly aroused when you're inside her, she won't love it—and you want her to love it, right?

5. Oh…did I mention that you tend to dive into the "target" too soon, ignoring the rest of her physical, mental, emotional and spiritual lusciousness? Take your time, guys, and enjoy the journey! The more fun she has getting there, the juicier it will be for you.

"For women the best aphrodisiacs are words. The G-spot is in the ears. He who looks for it below there is wasting his time."

ISABEL ALLENDE

FIVE THINGS THAT TURN HER ON

1. Discover all her favorite erogenous zones. Ears, toes, shoulders. Neck, belly, knees. Her pinky. The inside of her wrist . . . There's a whole lot of body there that isn't breast, nipple, pussy and ass. (I know: it can seem invisible sometimes!) Play with all of it!

2. Use words, ideas and fantasy. Her mind is her biggest erogenous zone: turn it on.

3. She wants romance and seduction. Give it to her.

4. Find out what her personal, private turn-ons are. Be willing to listen and have her show you. Real men ask for directions!

5. Keep your lovemaking inspired and spontaneous. Novelty, excitement and newness turn her on.

FIVE THINGS SHE NEEDS REASSURANCE ABOUT

1. That you love or care about her or at minimum, appreciate her company. (If you don't have any of these feelings for her, you might want to consider not having sex with her.)

2. That you love her body—shape, size, feel, smell, taste, capacities, everything! Almost all women in our culture have body image issues, even the ones you think are total hotties. Make a special point of reassuring her that you get off on how she looks, smells, tastes . . .

3. That you're dedicated to her pleasure.

4. That you especially love her yoni—its look, feel, taste and smell. Pussy-worship is a great aphrodisiac.

5. That she inspires desire in you. She wants you to want her!

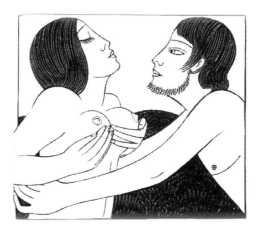

ERIC GILL, 1925

FIVE THINGS SHE WANTS FROM YOU

1. ATTUNED GIVING. Let your focus and direction be leavened by awareness and attunement. Initiate and direct not by dominating and going where you want, but by paying attention to her signals and taking her where she most wants to go. Give her exactly what she wants when she wants it by using your attention and presence in service to her pleasure. (Ultimately, her complete surrender to opening is exactly where you want to go, too!)

2. YOUR PRESENCE. If you don't show up, then who's that guy who's having sex with her?

3. CLEAN, CLEAR INTENTIONS AND INTEGRITY. Don't degrade yourself or her by manipulating or lying to her. Know what you want and speak your truth to her. If all you want is hot sex with no commitment, that's okay—tell her. That might be what she wants, too!

4. RELIABILITY AND DIRECTION. Women are "lunar," shifting and variable. They need a "solar" counterpoint—solid, steadfast male energy that doesn't tack with the breeze and can be counted on to provide clear focus and direction. You're the solid center; she dances around it (and if this sounds sexual, you're right!). Bring it on, Apollo!

5. YOUR HOT, STUDLY MASCULINE ENERGY. Be that demon lover, guys, but only when she's really ready—and ideally, begging for it!

So You Want to Be With a Sex Goddess!

UM, EXCUSE ME ... WHAT'S A "SEX GODDESS?"
I'm so glad you asked! My definition of a sex goddess is a woman who:

* Loves sex. (Really, really loves it!)

* Is wild and free.

* Is fun and playful.

* Is sexually and orgasmically proficient at a minimum, and is usually orgasmically abundant with expertise in all sex skills, including giving pleasure. If you really hit the jackpot (or maybe it's the jillpot), she may also be a shejaculator.

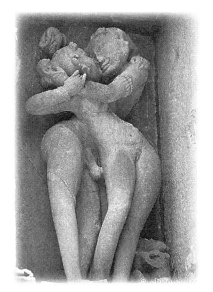

Temple Carvings—
Lakshman Temple, India

* Can look any way at all. You can't tell a sex goddess by her physical appearance, so don't get confused by the phony movie-star version. Sex goddesses come in all shapes and sizes. It's not how she looks, it's who she is!

* Totally mind-blowing sex (and other amazing kinds of blowing, too)

* The potential for transcendent connection and divine union

* Access to her glorious primal wildness

* Frequent and abundant ecstasy

* Did I mention the incredible sex?

If You Want A Sex Goddess In Your Bedroom ...

* Revere and adore her erotic energy, sexiness and passion.

* Call out her wildness and let her know you appreciate it thoroughly.

* Learn how to please her, and then be relentless in pursuing her pleasure.

* Meet her with your sacred, sexy god-self. One god(dess) is good. Two deities are divine!

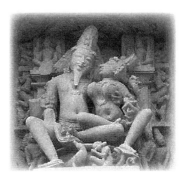

Temple carvings, India

Energy Essentials

There are two basic polarities of energy—feminine yin and masculine yang:

* Everyone has both qualities within them.

* Most people have a stronger, central, core energy and a secondary, balancing complementary energy.

* Most women have yin energy as their core, while most men have yang energy as their core.

* Sexual attraction is like the pull of two magnets—the opposite forces attract.

* We need to develop both our core and our complementary energy to be whole and healthy in ourselves and our relationships.

* The best sex happens when we have powerful currents of yin and yang flowing and forming circuits.

ABOUT YIN ENERGY

Yin sexual energy (usually the core energy of women):

*   Starts cool.

*   Is watery and fluid.

*   Often moves slowly.

*   Goes from the outer towards the inner.

*   Must pass through the other energy centers before it gets to the sex center in her crotch.

*   Is all about opening and receiving. Once she's received, the magic of transformation happens and she showers abundance and radiance back out.

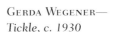

GERDA WEGENER— *Tickle, c. 1930*

ABOUT YANG ENERGY

Yang sexual energy (usually the core energy of men):

*   Starts hot.

*   Is fiery.

*   Is fast.

*   Starts in the sex center and can stay there or move outwards.

*   Is about penetrating or giving.

*   Is about initiation, focus, targeted goals and direction.

"Women need a reason to have sex. Men just need a place."

BILLY CRYSTAL

THE PLAY OF YIN AND YANG

When yin and ying are interacting:

•   The energies create an erotic circuit that can travel within an individual or between people.

•   Inside our self, we're always dancing with both energies, balancing our power.

•   The secondary or complementary energy balances, leavens, mitigates and expands our core energy.

Yin energy:

* Starts outside her body, in her relationships and in the context. It needs to feel safe and connected (see *Five Things You Need to Know About Women*, above).

* Moves inward, starting from outside her, then proceeding to her edges and slowly moving towards her center.

* Is like a pot of cool water that takes time to come to a boil—and only does so when the proper (or improper!) heat is applied. The arousal energy needs time to accumulate in her genitals.

* Can be easily distracted, drained or blocked.

* Deeply desires to open and receive, to surrender fully. And to explode in grateful, ecstatic showers.

SUZUKI HARUNOBU— *Shunga, c. 1750*

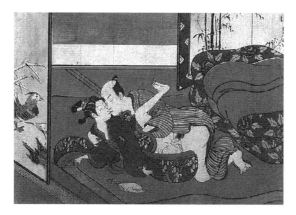

ALIGNING YIN & YANG AROUSAL

* Yang arousal is fast. Yin is slow. You're better off slowing down to her pace than trying to get her to speed up to yours.

* The more attention you give to her pleasure, the more she'll love sex and the more she'll want to have it with you. What goes around comes around (and if she's a sex goddess, often!)

* Breathe together—it helps align the energies.

* Share sounds of pleasure and passion—ditto!

* Communicate with words, gestures, body language, looks and energy.

Let's Get Physical

* Start by focusing on connecting.

* Wake up her whole body, beginning with the non-sexual parts.

* Proceed slowly—take your time getting to the "good stuff.'" Don't rush headlong (or with any body parts) into her hot spots. (Like they say: it's all good!)

* This doesn't mean the rhythm of your touch should always be slow. Vary the energy and pacing. Be inventive, attuned and present.

* Tease, tantalize, coax, entice and titillate. Help her want more, not less. Better to have her longing for you to touch her genitals than thinking, "There he is with his hand in my crotch, and I'm not even turned on yet!"

* Don't play with her tender bits (genitals and nipples) until she's already turned on. Play with that stuff after she's aroused, not as the way to get her turned on. (This is a prime example of how different she is from you!)

GERDA WEGENER—
c. 1930

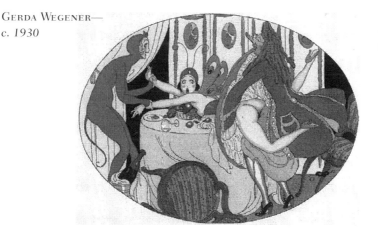

*"For flavor, instant sex will never supersede
the stuff you have to peel and cook."*

QUENTIN CRISP

* Focus on her breasts, ass and genitals too much and too soon. Have I mentioned that you tend to zoom in on the targets and dive into her crevices before she's ready? Cut it out. It's giving your whole gender a bad name as impatient and immature.

* Be inconsiderate and selfish, with too much focus on your pleasure. Remember, ladies come first!

* Behave in a way that will trigger fear, anger, resentment or anxiety in her. Her sexual energy needs to pass through all her other energetic centers before it reaches her crotch. Any of these emotions will block it from getting there.

* Bring to the bedroom stinky smells, rough stubble, ragged, sharp fingernails . . . need I go on? Cleanliness may not be next to godliness, but it will certainly help you get next to goddesses!

* Be boring and predictable. Don't "fuck by numbers," even if it worked great the last time. There is no one right way. Do you want her dozing off because she's been down this road way too often before?

* Act in a way that causes her to feel unsafe or transgressed.

How To Touch Her So She Melts

* Honor and respect her boundaries carefully and utterly. Check in if you aren't sure about something, and keep checking in if you have any reason whatsoever to believe you may be crossing a line.

* Touch transmits intention, so make sure yours are clear, honest and welcome. On that note, if you're just touching a peripheral part because "you have to" to get to the crotch, she'll know it and it won't feel good.

* Bring your utter presence and awareness into your fingertips, or whatever else is making contact. Don't just touch—*feel*.

* Pay attention to her signals of opening (she likes it) or closing (she doesn't).

* Learn the four languages of touch—therapeutic, nurturing, sensual and sexual. Dance among them. Use them all.

* This is the First Commandment of lovemaking: she wants to be aroused before you touch her genitals. Premature pussy play is a no-fun no-no. She's got an arousal stairway—sort of a ten-step program. Wait until mid-level arousal (step five) or better before heading for the juicy bits.

* Visualize her body as having a series of concentric zones starting with her energy fields and proceeding from there to her non-erogenous zones, her erogenous zones and her genitals. Start at the outer zones and

ANONYMOUS—*Daphnis and Chloe, c. 1890*

slowly work your way toward the pussy. During her early-stage arousal, avoid the more sensitive areas such as her ass-crack and nipples. Until she's at medium arousal, steer clear of the crevices.

* Don't proceed to the next inner zone until she signals that she wants you to. Only approach the genitals after you've spent a fair amount of time in the outer zones. Cruise the border and work the energy fields. Teasing is good!

* Never, ever go pushing and shoving your way into her most sacred space. We *hate* that. Pay attention to her opening to you or her closing away from you! If she has her legs closed, it means she doesn't want you going there. When she's ready, she'll open to your touch. Wait until you're invited to enter, or even better, begged!

* A woman's signs of high arousal are intense breathing, more sound and body movement, all of which increase as arousal builds. At the same time, every woman is a bit different. Learn her particular signs so you'll know where she is on her arousal journey. And remember: vaginal lubrication is an indicator of early arousal, not "Stick it in me, Big Guy!" readiness. Don't assume that just because she's wet, she's primed to be entered. If you aren't sure where she is in her arousal journey—ask!

"Anything worth doing is worth doing slowly."
MAE WEST

* Remember: awaken her whole body and get her excitement to the moderate range before you head for the genital region.

* Play with the energy fields around the breasts, ass and pussy before you make contact. It makes us really want you to touch it!

* Begin by going to the vicinity of your target. Play with the nearby body parts, like the thighs, butt checks and belly. Hang out in the neighborhood until she's begging for more focused genital attention.

* Tease her. Almost go there, skim and pass by, advance and retreat— make her crazy with wanting. Let her wanting precede your giving!

PLAYING WITH PUSSY

* Start with the "yard." This is the outside of the vulva, the area that is covered by hair and regular skin. You can stroke, pet, rub, squeeze and play with her entire vulva from the yard. Stay there until her arousal level is moderate (six) or higher. By pressing down firmly on the whole vulva, you stimulate her vestibular bulbs, which can become big puffy mounds of erectile tissue.

* Next comes the "porch." This is the delicate mucous membrane area between the outer lips, but not yet inside her pussy. This is a *no-friction zone*. Mucosa is tissue that is designed to be wet, so only touch it wetly. Slip and slide here with lots of lube, saliva or some of her pussy juice.

* The clitoris can be accessed from the yard or the porch. Always begin with indirect and diffuse stimulation. Be gentle, darling! And don't poke.

* Don't enter the inner sanctum of her vagina until her arousal level is high (eight or more). You can ruin all that fine work you've done if you try to slip in a finger (or anything else) too soon. You'll know it's right if it feels as if she's sucking you in. When that happens, it's brain-basement girl-talk for "Oh yeah, give it to me!"

* When you enter her with your fingers, do it consciously and carefully. Usually, slowly is better than a quick deep thrust (unless instructed otherwise!) Take your time, explore and play with all of the erectile structures that are around and just inside the entrance.

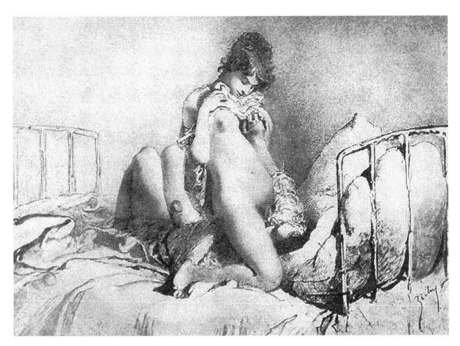

MIHALY ZICHY, c. 1880

FACILITATING HER ORGASM

* Help her own her pleasure. If she doesn't pet her own pussy, encourage her to do so.

* Ask her to show you how she makes herself come. Practice till you can do it just the way she likes it.

* Encourage her to breathe deeply, release her sound, and move her body inside with her pelvic muscles and outside with her pelvis and spine.

* Pay attention and be utterly attuned to her signals of what's working and what's not. Feminine energy fluxes and shifts, so what worked last week may not be as effective this week.

* When you are doing something that catches her rhythm and is moving her into higher and higher arousal, *don't stop or change*. Keep doing what you're doing. Don't get harder or faster or move from that spot. Keep it up (I mean, keep going). Be relentless!

* Egg her on, be her coach, cheer her wildness, and tell her how sexy she looks, sounds and feels. Encourage, goad and applaud her. Root for her. Buoy her up. Be her best (and most studly) cheerleader, ever!

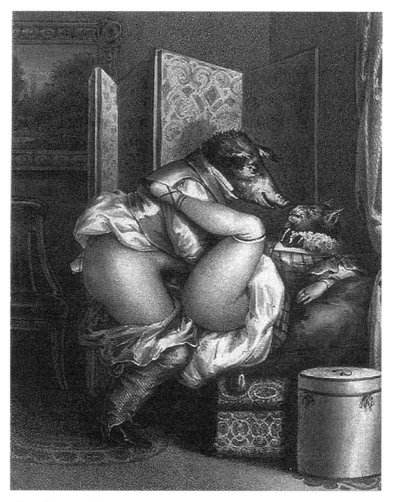

JEAN-JACQUES GRANDVILLE

FUCKING SO SHE LOVES IT

* Absolutely, positively don't put anything inside her until she's at high arousal (eight or higher). If you want to play it really safe, wait until she's had her first orgasm.

* Enter gently. While variety is important and the occasional first fast full thrust in can be delicious at the perfect moment, in general, enter slowly, feeling your way in. Never forget that you're in someone else's body!

* Once inside, take your time. I mean, really, guys: do you have anything better to do? Play with all the exciting areas of her arousal network. Don't think you need to be in all the way every moment: you can use your head (of your cock, that is) to explore the opening, too.

* *Friction is not your friend or hers.* Use plenty of lube and apply it repeatedly, especially at the vaginal opening.

* There's a time for wild monkey-fucking and a time for a cooler groove. Learn the fine art of friction-free fucking, when you rock your hips rather than pump your loins. One of the benefits of the frictionless approach is that her vagina won't get irritated and sore, so you can keep going longer. This is especially important if you're circumcised—no sleeve means more friction.

> *"Fifty percent of the women in this country are not having orgasms. If that were true of the male population, it would be declared a national emergency."*
>
> MARGO ST. JAMES

* Keep it interesting. Use a variety of patterns and rhythms. Use short strokes and long ones and patterns of both. Be bold, be gentle. Don't go pounding away unless she's at high-level arousal and responding well to your deep thrusts. Use angled strokes, subtle twisting motions, your pelvic floor muscles, and small movements of your sacrum. Try for gliding, pulsing, rocking motions, especially with your cock deep inside. As always, be super-attuned to what's working for her.

* Use clitoral stimulation while fucking. It will increase her arousal and pleasure. Use fingers (yours or hers) or a handy vibrator.

* Learn to channel your sexual energy so that you can ejaculate when the moment's right for you both.

* If you come before she does, it doesn't mean the sex is over. Be a gentleman and serve her until she's fully satisfied.

> *"If a woman has to choose between catching a fly ball and saving an infant's life, she will choose to save the infant's life without even considering if there are men on base."*
>
> DAVE BARRY

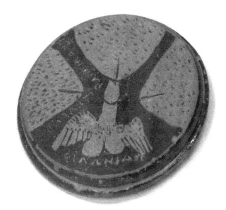

WINGED PHALLUS—GREEK, C. 460-425 BC

Never mind what Yogi Berra said: it ain't over till *after* it's over:

* Once you've come, you may want to just drift off to sleep. Before you do, though, do yourself and your sweetie a favor. Say three nice things. "Man, that was hot!" "I love how your pussy tastes!" Or even: "I love you" (but only if it's true). You'll have created the after-sex connection she wants—then you can go into your post-ejaculatory coma.

* Snuggle and cuddle. (C'mon, you know you like it, too.)

* Ask her what she loved and what worked to really get her going (and coming). Remember those tricks for next time!

* Tell her some things that you loved and that you thought were really sexy. Let her know what turned you on! She'll remember and give it to you again—and it's another opportunity to let her know how sizzling she was.

* Thank her. Everyone appreciates gratitude.

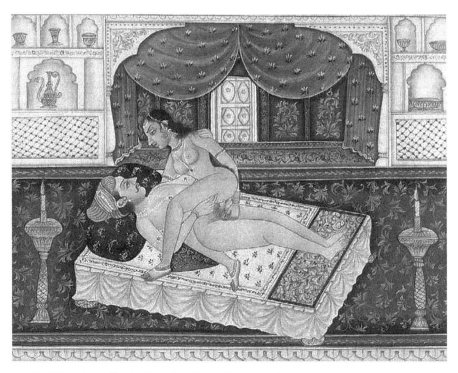

Erotic Miniature Illustrating the Kama Sutra, India

Thanks, Guys, That Was Great!

SO NOW WE'VE COME TO THE END of your short course. A condensed version isn't the whole thing, of course. If you aspire to be a fabulous lover, you'll probably need to at least skim the rest of the book. At a minimum, read the HOT TIPS FOR GUYS sidebars, which will expand on the information in this chapter. I also suggest that you study the chapters on female anatomy, so you can discover where all her yummy bits are. In those pages, you'll find useful suggestions for making all of those parts very happy—and the homework's really fun, too!

Of course, if you really want to be a world-class lover, you'll need more information than you'll get from reading this chapter and the HOT TIPS. Even reading the middle section and discovering where all the juicy parts are is not enough. If you aspire to true erotic virtuosity, it will help to read the whole book. In addition, and I know it will devastate you to hear this, you'll have to practice. This means having a lot of sex (including with yourself). You'll also need to practice the skills of the body, heart, mind and spirit—and relationship skills like communication, too.

If you do this, your life will become immeasurably richer, hotter and more connected. You'll reap all the benefits of great sex, including aerobic exercise, meditative brain-states, relaxation and rejuvenation, amazing intimacy and—did I forget to mention this?—mind-blowing pleasure.

Ultimately, sex is about connecting—about channeling erotic energy and gaining access to the life force. As a man, you're probably drawn to do that by connecting to your opposite polarity—the great, magical and compelling force of the feminine. Honor your desire. Follow your attraction with integrity and respect using your masculine presence, power and skill. When you revere all the manifestations of the feminine—in women, in yourself and in the world—you'll tap into the mother lode, the source of everything, the gateway to the universe. This book has laid out maps to this sacred, wild, erotic feminine realm. Come explore! There's treasure awaiting discovery . . . .

"The Eternal Feminine draws us upward."

GOETHE

Appendices

Anatomy Illustration Notes and Credits

All anatomy and incidental illustrations are by the author, Sheri Winston, unless otherwise noted.

ANATOMY ILLUSTRATION ORIENTATION

These indicators are based on the standard anatomical position for human anatomy, which is standing erect, forward facing:

- FRONT VIEW: As if you're looking straight at the woman.

- SIDE VIEW (also known as the medial mid-sagittal cross-section): As if you're looking at the woman, from the side, usually as if they were sectioned (sliced in half) and opened for view.

- THREE-QUARTER VIEW: As if you're looking at the person from an angle in between the front and the side, like you're looking at the front point of the hip.

In addition, many images in this book utilize an additional perspective:

- BOTTOM VIEW: As if the woman were lying on her back with her legs spread open, and you were looking at her crotch. (Unofficially called the split beaver view.)

ADDITIONAL USEFUL ANATOMICAL TERMS

- SUPERIOR—toward the head

- INFERIOR—away from the head

- ANTERIOR—the front of the body or body part

- POSTERIOR—the back of the body or body part

- MEDIAL—toward the midline that divides left and right

- LATERAL—to the side away from the midline

- SUPERFICIAL—on top, or towards the surface

- DEEP – inside, towards the center

About the Author

SHERI WINSTON CNM, RN, BSN, LMT is a sex teacher whose classes and workshops for men and women are celebrated for their fun, non-threatening character and superb content. Winston's unique perspective, which she calls Wholistic Sexuality™, is derived from decades of experience as a certified nurse-midwife, gynecology practitioner, registered nurse, holistic healer, childbirth educator, massage therapist and student of the esoteric erotic arts. She is the executive director of the Intimate Arts Center (IntimateArtsCenter.com).

My Story

I WAS BLESSED AT THE AGE OF TWENTY by my calling to be a midwife (which I like to call the second oldest profession). I spent the next two decades on my knees in front of the amazing altar of birth.

While my primary path was always the practice of midwifery (with some holistic gynecology as well), I've also been a teacher. No matter what else I was doing, I always taught classes of some kind alongside my main work.

To be a good practitioner and teacher requires one to always be learning. I went through many years of formal education, receiving certifications in massage therapy and childbirth education, and degrees in nursing, gynecology and midwifery. Along with the birthing arts, I studied and practiced holistic natural healing (especially herbalism, energywork, guided visualization, sound healing and various forms of touch and bodywork).

My greatest teacher was the birth process itself. I have been granted the gift of being present at over 500 births—each truly a miracle. Most were natural births, beautiful, powerful and exquisitely choreographed by Mother Nature's ancient inherent wisdom.* Being present for those births allowed me to see life's template—inescapably up-close and personal. I worked hard to learn how to serve that power rather than interfere with it. As a midwife, I viewed it as my job to honor and facilitate the natural process. While I occasionally needed to use my medical knowledge and skill to actually do something for mom or baby, my main task was to help the woman connect to her inherent knowledge about

---

* By natural birth, I mean that the mother didn't use medications, that she was active and at choice about how to give birth, and that there was as little interference as possible with the biological template. These were home or birth center experiences, since it's almost impossible to have a natural birth experience in a hospital. Unfortunately, the joyous and potentially ecstatic experience of natural birth is quite rare in our culture.

how to bring life into this world. Women have their own intuitive wisdom about how to navigate the profound and primal rite of passage that is birth—I was there to help them find and use that knowledge.

Spending twenty years serving the power of birth turned out to be the best possible apprenticeship I could have for being a sex teacher. My second calling, which I launched about a decade ago, has taken me deeper into the same mystery. Following my passion for birth, I have traced that miracle back to its roots in the perfect magic of sex.

It was the birth process that taught me much of what I learned about how to have great sex, although at first I didn't realize it. For years, I taught women how to breathe themselves into an altered state; how to surrender to the tide of labor; how to release their sound and use it to open themselves; and how to use their pelvic muscles as well as their mind to facilitate the birth process. I helped women get in touch with their innate wisdom and showed them how to use their inner tools to cooperate with the natural process.

Unwittingly, I had incorporated these same skills and practices into my own increasingly fabulous sex life. Once I become aware that I'd been unconsciously using these techniques, I decided it was time to start learning and practicing them purposefully. I now understood that I'd been on a learning journey about sexuality for my whole life, and that if I made the study of it a conscious practice, the sex would only get better. This is what I did, and what was already fabulous sex became totally mind-blowing.

I have always loved to learn, and sex has always been a favorite subject for this avid scholar. I've been an ardent student of eros as far back as I can remember. Curiosity probably propelled me more than desire when I began my explorations. Now, both the lust to learn and the other kind of eros fuel my desire to experience ever-deeper levels of ecstasy, intimacy and freedom.

I've been very blessed in my life. I feel profoundly honored to have been granted access to so many awe-inspiring birth experiences. Over the years, my sexuality, intimate relationships and professional work have come together to enable me to have amazing sex and relationships. It's not only my joy but my responsibility to take the gifts I've received and give them back so others can benefit.

This book is a distillation of what I've had the extraordinary good fortune to learn. It is my service, my privilege and my joy to share it with you. Thank you for receiving it!

Bibliography

Anand, Margo. *The Art of Sexual Ecstasy.* New York: Tarcher/Putnam, 1989.

Andresen, Gail L. & Weinhold, Barry K. *Connective Bargaining.* Englewood Cliffs, NJ: Prentice Hall, 1981.

Angier, Natalie. *Woman: An Intimate Geography.* New York: Anchor Books, 2000.

Baker, Jeannine Parvati & Baker, Frederick & Slayton, Tamara. *Conscious Conception.* Sevier, UT: Freestone Publishing, 1986.

Barbach, Lonnie. *Sharing Sexual Intimacy.* New York: Signet, 1984.

Barstow, Anne Llewellyn. *Witchcraze.* San Francisco: Harper Collins, 1995.

Belenky, Mary Field & Clinchy, Blythe McVicker & Goldberger, Nancy Rule & Tarule, Jill Mattuck *Women's Ways of Knowing.* New York: Basic Books, 1986.

Bidloo, Govard. *Ontleding des menschelyken lichaams.* Amsterdam: Weduwe van Joannes van Someren, et al., 1690

Blank, Joanie. *Femalia.* San Francisco: Down There Press, 1993.

Blonna, Richard & Levitan, Jean. *Healthy Sexuality.* Englewood, CO: Morton Publishing Company, 2000.

Blue, Violet. *The Ultimate Guide to Fellatio.* San Francisco: Cleis Press, 2002.

Blue, Violet *The Ultimate Guide to Cunnilingus.* San Francisco: Cleis Press, 2002.

Bodansky, Steve & Bodansky, Vera. *Extended Massive Orgasm.* Alameda, CA: Hunter House, 2000.

Bonheim, Jalaja. *Aphrodite's Daughter.* New York: Fireside, Simon & Schuster, 1997.

Boston Women's Health Book Collective. *Our Bodies, Ourselves.* New York: A Touchstone Book, Simon & Schuster, 2005.

Brauer, Alan P. & Brauer, Donna. *ESO* (*Extended Sexual Orgasm).* New York: Warner Books, 1983.

Calais-Germain, Blandine. *The Female Pelvis.* Seattle: Eastland Press, 2003.

Camphausen, Rufus C., *The Encycopedia of Sacred Sexuality.* Rochester, VT: Inner Traditions, 1999.

Camphausen, Rufus C. *The Yoni.* Rochester, VT: Inner Traditions, 1996.

Carellas, Barbara & Sprinkle, Annie. *Urban Tantra.* Celestial Arts, 2007.

Chalker, Rebecca. *The Clitoral Truth.* New York: Seven Stories Press, 2000.

Chia, Mantak & Chia, Maneewan. *Healing Love Through the Tao: Cultivating Female Sexual Energy.* Huntington, NY: Healing Tao, 1986.

Chronicle Books. *Going Down.* (compilation) San Francisco: Chronicle, 1998.

Comfort, Alex. *The Joy of Sex.* New York: Crown Publishers, 1972.

Comfort, Alex. *More Joy of Sex.* New York: Crown Publishers, 1974.

Cousin, Jehan. *Livre de pourtraiture.* Paris: Jean Leclerc, 1608.

Dale, Cyndi. *The Subtle Body.* Boulder: Sounds True, 2009.

Davis, Elizabeth. *Women's Sexual Passages.* Alameda, CA: Hunter House, 2000.

Davis, Elizabeth & Leonard, Carol. *The Women's Wheel of Life.* New York: Penguin Arkana, 1997.

Deida, David. *Intimate Communion*. Deerfield Beach, FL: Health Communications, Inc., 1995.

Deida, David *It's a Guy Thing*. Deerfield Beach, FL: Health Communications, Inc., 1995.

Deida, David *The Way of the Superior Man*. Austin, TX: Plexus, 1997.

Deida, David *Blue Truth*. Boulder, CO: Sounds True, Inc. 2005

DeRopp, Robert S. *Sex Energy*. New York: Delacorte Press, 1969.

Devi, Kamala. *The Eastern Way of Love*. New York: Fireside, 1985.

Diagram Group, The. *Sex: A User's Manual*. New York: Perigee Books, 1981

Dodson, Betty. *Orgasms for Two*. New York: Harmony, 2002.

Dodson, Betty. *Sex For One*. New York: Crown Publishers, 1987.

Doolittle, Ducky. *Sex With the Lights On*. Da Capo Press, 2006.

Douglas, Marcia & Douglas, Lisa. *The Sex You Want*. New York: Marlowe & Co., 2002.

Douglas, Nik & Slinger, Penny. *Sexual Secrets*. Rochester, VT: Destiny Books, 1979.

Dunas, Felice. *Passion Play*. Riverhead Trade, 1998.

Dürer, Albrecht. *Vier Bücher von menschlicher Proportion*. Nuremberg: Hieronymus Formschneyder, 1528.

Easton, Dossie & Hardy, Janet W. *The Ethical Slut: A Practical Guide to Polyamory, Open Relationships & Other Adventures*. Celestial Arts, 2009.

Ehrenreich, Barbara & English, Dierdre. *For Her Own Good*. Garden City, NY: Anchor Books, 1979.

England, Pam. *Birthing from Within*. Partera Press, 1998.

Eisler, Riane. *Sacred Pleasure*. San Francisco: Harper, 1995.

Federation of Feminist Women's Health Centers. *A New View of a Woman's Body*. Los Angeles: Feminist Health Press, 1991.

Firefox, LaSara. *Sexy Witch*. Woodbury, MN: Llewellyn, 2005.

Fisher, Helen. *Why We Love*. New York: Henry Holt & Co., 2004.

Frankel, Carl. *Out of the Labyrinth*. Rhinebeck, NY: Monkfish, 2004.

Franklin, Eric. *Pelvic Power*. Hightstown, NJ: Elysian Editions, Princeton Book Co., 2003.

Frye, Anne. *Healing Passage: A Suturing Manual for Midwives* (4th ed.). Labrys Press, 1991.

Goddard, Jamie & Brungardt, Kurt. *Lesbian Sex Secrets for Men*. New York: Plume, 2000.

Gray, Henry. *Anatomy, Descriptive and Surgical, 1901 Edition*. Philadelphia, London: Running Press, 1974.

Haddon, Genia Pauli. *Uniting Sex Self & Spirit*. Scotland, CT: Plus Publications, 1993.

Heart, Mikaya. *When the Earth Moves: Women and Orgasm*. Berkeley: Celestial Arts, 1998.

Henderson, Julie. *The Lover Within*. Barrytown, NY: Station Hill, 1987.

Hendrix, Harville *Getting the Love You Want*. New York: HarperPerennial, 1990.

Hooper, Anne. *Great Sex Guide*. New York: DK Publishing, 1999.

Joannides, Paul. *Guide to Getting it On!* (3rd ed.) Saline, MI: Goofy Foot Press, 2000.

Judith, Anodea. *Chakra: Wheels of Life.* Laurier Books, 2004.

Kitzinger, Sheila. *Woman's Experience of Sex.* Toronto: G.P. Putnam & Sons, 1983.

Laqueur, Thomas. *Making Sex.* Cambridge, MA.: Harvard Univ. Press, 1990.

Levay, Simon. *The Sexual Brain.* Cambridge, MA: MIT Press, 1993.

Lewis, Thomas & Amini, Fari & Lannon, Richard. *A General Theory of Love.* New York: Random House, 2000.

Lichtman, Ronnie & Papera, Susan. *Gynecology: Well-woman Care.* Norwalk, CT: Appleton & Lange, 1990.

McCary, James L. *Human Sexuality.* Princeton: Van Nostrand, 1967.

Masters, William H. & Johnson, Virginia E. & Kolodny, Robert C. *Masters and Johnson on Sex and Human Loving.* Boston: Little Brown, 1986.

Mellen, Sidney L. W. *The Evolution of Love.* San Francisco: Freeman, 1981.

Meyer, Cheryl L. *The Wandering Uterus.* New York: New York University Press, 1997.

Montagu, Ashley. *Touching.* New York: Harper, 1986.

Mumfor, Dr. Jonn. *Ecstasy Through Tantra.* St. Paul, MN:Llewellyn Publications, 1988.

Muscio, Inga. *Cunt: A Declaration of Independence.* New York: Seal Press, 2002.

Myss, Caroline. *Energy Anatomy.* Boulder: Sounds True, 2001.

Nash, Elizabeth. *Plaisirs d'Amour.* New York: Harper Collins, 1995.

Netter, Frank. *The CIBA Collection of Medical Illustrations Vol 2 Reproductive System.* New York: CIBA Pharmaceutical Co. 1965.

Offit, Avodah K. *The Sexual Self.* New York: Congdon & Weed, 1983.

Paget, Lou. *Orgasms.* New York: Broadway Books, 2004.

Pert, Candace B. *Molecules of Emotion: Why You Feel the Way You Feel.* New York: Scribner, 1997.

Ramsdale, David and Ellen. *Sexual Energy Ecstasy.* New York: Bantam, 1993.

Rama, Swami & Ballentine, Rudolph & Hymes, Alan. *Science of Breath: A Practical Guide.* Honesdale, PA: Himalayan Institute Press, 1998.

Ratey, John J. *A User's Guide to the Brain.* New York: Vintage, 2002.

Saraswati, Sunyata & Avinasha, Bodhi. *Jewel in the Lotus.* Ipsalu Publishing, 2006.

Savage, Linda E. *Reclaiming Goddess Sexuality.* Carlsbad, CA: Hay House, 1999.

Scantling, Sandra R. *Extraordinary Sex Now.* New York: Doubleday, 1998.

Scantling, Sandra R. & Browder, Sue. *Ordinary Women, Extraordinary Sex.* New York: Dutton, 1993.

Schlossberg, Leon & Zuidema, George D. *The Johns Hopkins Atlas of Human Functional Anatomy.* Baltimore: Johns Hopkins University Press, 1977.

Sevely, Josephine Lowndes. *Eve's Secret.* New York: Random House, 1987.

Singer, Katie *Honoring Our Cycles.* Winona Lake, IN: New Trends, 2006.

Smith, Bradley. *Erotic Art of the Masters: The 18th, 19th and 20th Centuries.* New York: Galley Press

Schnarch, David. *Passionate Marriage*. W.W. Norton & Co., 2009.

Spiegel, Adriaan van & Casseri, Giulio *De Humani corporis fabrica libri decem*. Venice: Evangelista Deuchino, 1627.

Sprinkle, Annie. *Dr. Sprinkle's Spectacular Sex*. Tarcher, 2005.

Strong, Brian & DeVault, Christine & Sayad, Barbara Werner. *Human Sexuality: Diversity in Contemporary America*. (3rd ed.) Mountain View, CA: Mayfield Publishing, 1999.

Strong, Brian & DeVault, Christine & Sayad, Barbara Werner. *Core Concepts in Human Sexuality*. Mountain View, CA: Mayfield Publishing, 1996.

Stubbs, Kenneth Ray. *The Essential Tantra*. New York: Tarcher/Putnam, 1993.

Sundahl, Deborah. *Female Ejaculation & the G-Spot*. Alameda, CA: Hunter House, 2003.

Tannahill, Reay. *Sex in History* Briarcliff Manor, NY: Stein and Day, 1980.

Tannen, Deborah *You Just Don't Understand*. New York: Ballantine, 1990.

Tannen, Deborah *That's Not What I Meant!* New York: Ballantine, 1986.

Taylor, Patricia *Expanded Orgasm: Soar to Ecstasy at Your Lover's Every Touch*. Naperville, IL: Sourcebooks, 2002.

Twala w/ Smith, Robb. *Sacred Sex*. San Rafael, CA: Mandala, 1993.

Valverde de Amusco, Juan *Anatomia del corpo humano*.
Rome: Salamanca and Antonio Lafrey, 1560.

Waxman, Jamye. *Getting Off: A Woman's Guide to Masturbation*. Emeryville, CA: Seal Press, 2007.

Index

A

Accelerating breath, 189
Acid-alkaline balance (pH), 120
Adept stage of sexual learning, 52
Allende, Isabel, 175, 239
Allen, Woody, 20, 171
Altered spaces, 205
Altered state of consciousness, 12, 13
Alter ego, 202
Amrita, 134–135, 230–231
Anal sex. *See* Anus
Anatomy. *See* Female genital anatomy,
    knowledge of
Angelou, Maya, 79
Anterior sponge. *See* Urethral sponge
Anus, 136–139
    arousal of, 138–139
    defined, 137
    exploration of, 136
    hygiene of, 138
Anxiety, 218
Areola, 141–142, 144
Aristotle, 164
Arousal
    anatomy of, 144–153
    of anus, 138–139
    of breasts, 144
    of clitoris, 106
    high, 84
    levels of, 145
    medium, 84
    of nerves within vagina, 127
    non, 84
    orgasms with male, 228–230
    stages of, 84
    ten-step process for, 13–15
    trances, 12–13, 14
    of urethral sponge, 114
    of uterus, 123–124
    of vagina, 119
    of vestibular bulbs, 111
    See also Sexual arousal
Arousal trance, 12–13, 14
Attention, 172–174
Attitude, 205
Auden, W. H., 198
Aural sex, 190–193
Aurelius, Marcus, 162, 188
Awareness, 172–174

B

Baby talk, 30
Bacterial vaginosis (BV), 120
Bartholins glands, 133
Beauvoir, Simone de, 66
Berra, Yogi, 251

Big draw, 189
Bladder, 125
Bleeding time, 154–155
Bly, Robert, 44
Body, acceptance of, 165–166
Body techniques, 187
    combination of all, 197, 203–204
    defined, 161
Bonaparte, Marie, 107
Bottom sponge, 116
Boundaries, 5, 31, 33, 74
Breast-feeding, 142–143, 152–153
Breasts, 141–157
    anatomy of, 141–142
    arousal of, 144
    defined, 141
Breath augmentation, 189
Breath awareness practice, 189
Breathing techniques, 185–189
    practicing basic, 189
Buddha, Gautama, 17, 183, 235
Bulbocavernosus, 148
Byrne, Robert, 68

C

Candida, 120
Capillaries, 101–103
Capote, Truman, 200
Carter, Angela, 46
Ceremony, 205, 208–210
Cervix, 121
Chakras system, 15, 221–223
Chi, 59
Christianity, 25, 40
Clitoral body. *See* Clitoral shaft
Clitoral corpus. *See* Clitoral shaft
Clitoral glands, 105
Clitoral head, 105-106
Clitoral hood, 90, 92
Clitoral legs, 105, 106–107
Clitoral shaft, 105–106, 107
    defined, 107
    exploration of, 105–106
    rolling technique of, 107
Clitoris, 35–36, 94–96, 105–108
    anatomy of, 105, 144
    arousal of, 106
    defined, 104
    exploration of, 105–108
    techniques for touching, 108
Compassion, 182
Conception, 156
Connection pattern, 197
Core yin and yang
    explained, 64–65, 69
    suppressing, 72
    uncomplemented, 71
Courage, 170